The Cytology of Soft Tissue Tumours

Monographs in Clinical Cytology

Vol. 16

Series Editor

Svante R. Orell Kent Town

KARGER

The Cytology of Soft Tissue Tumours

Måns Åkerman, Patologisk/Cytologisk Klinik, Lund
Henryk A. Domanski, Patologisk/Cytologisk Klinik, Lund

Including contributions by

Anders Rydholm, Ortopedisk Klinik, Lund
Brigitta Carlén, Patologisk/Cytologisk Klink, Lund

78 figures, 78 in color, and 10 tables, 2003

KARGER

Basel · Freiburg · Paris · London · New York ·
Bangalore · Bangkok · Singapore · Tokyo · Sydney

The Cytology of Soft Tissue Tumours

Dr. Måns Åkerman
Dr. Henryk A. Domanski
Patologisk/Cytologisk Klinik
Universitetssjukhuset
SE–221 85 Lund
Tel. +46 46 17 35 10, Fax +46 46 14 33 07
E-Mail mans.akerman@skane.se; henryk.Domanski@pat.lu.se

Library of Congress Cataloging-in-Publication Data

Åkerman, Måns.
The cytology of soft tissue tumours / Måns Åkerman, Henryk A. Domanski; in collaboration with Anders Rydholm, Brigitta Carlén.
p. ; cm. – (Monographs in clinical cytology ; vol. 16)
Includes bibliographical references and index.
ISBN 3–8055–7594–7
1. Soft tissue tumors–Cytodiagnosis. I. Domanski, Henryk A. II. Title. III. Series.
[DNLM: 1. Cytological Techniques. 2. Soft Tissue Neoplasms. WD 375 A314c 2003]
RC280.S66A347 2003
616.99′207582–dc21 2003054510

Bibliographic Indices. This publication is listed in bibliographic services, including Current Contents® and Index Medicus.

Drug Dosage. The authors and the publisher have exerted every effort to ensure that drug selection and dosage set forth in this text are in accord with current recommendations and practice at the time of publication. However, in view of ongoing research, changes in government regulations, and the constant flow of information relating to drug therapy and drug reactions, the reader is urged to check the package insert for each drug for any change in indications and dosage and for added warnings and precautions. This is particularly important when the recommended agent is a new and/or infrequently employed drug.

P.O. Box, CH–4009 Basel (Switzerland)
Printed in Switzerland on acid-free paper by
Reinhardt Druck, Basel
www.karger.com
ISBN 3–8055–7594–7

Contents

Preface

The cytological diagnosis of soft tissue tumours, based on fine needle aspirates, has been debated and at times discouraged except in the diagnosis of lipoma. Soft tissue tumours are relatively rare in spite of the fact that more than 100 benign subtypes, over 50 variants of sarcoma and a number of 'border-line' entities have been described. Individual cytopathologists are thus not likely to encounter many of the less common variants of soft tissue tumours during their training and may only occasionally needle them in their later practice. It has been strongly recommended that the primary morphological diagnosis of malignant soft tissue tumours as well as other investigations and treatment should be performed at multidisciplinary centres. In practice, however, it is not possible to refer all patients with soft tissue tumours to a musculoskeletal tumour centre for primary work-up. Tumours are usually considered to be suspicious if they are large (>5 cm) or deep-seated (inter-or intramuscular). This implies that the management of the majority of soft tissue tumours is undertaken in general hospitals.

The use of special diagnostic methods has led to greater accuracy in histopathological diagnosis in this tumour group. The use of ancillary methods is also, no doubt, necessary in many cases when fine needle aspiration (FNA) and cytodiagnosis is used in primary diagnosis, making surgical biopsy unnecessary. As has repeatedly been demonstrated in other tumour entities, the use of FNA instead of surgical biopsy or core needle biopsy offers a number of advantages when used in the primary diagnosis of soft tissue tumours.

The purpose of this book is to facilitate the cytological evaluation of FNA smears from soft tissue tumours and suggest cytological criteria for a histotype diagnosis. The aim is foremost to describe and illustrate the most common entities and those rare tumours where cytological features have been described in case-reports and in small series.

The diagnostic use of ancillary methods is also discussed and illustrated.

The selection of entities which will be presented, their diagnostic features and differential diagnostic considerations are mainly based on the experience with FNA in the primary diagnosis of soft tissue tumours in patients referred to the Musculoskeletal Tumour Centre, University Hospital, Lund, Sweden over a 25-year period. Cases from the soft tissue tumour registry of the Scandinavian Sarcoma Group (a multidisciplinary association with members from all Nordic countries) have also been used. The illustrations have been culled from cases in the files of the Department of Pathology and Cytology, Lund University Hospital, which now contains smears from more than 3,000 soft tissue tumours needled between 1972 and 2002.

Måns Åkerman
Henryk A. Domanski

Acknowledgements

The authors thank Dr. Svante Orell, Clinpath Laboratories, Adelaide, Australia for his help. Svante Orell is the scientific editor for the series *Monographs in Clinical Cytology* and his comments and revisions of the text have been invaluable. We thank Dr. Walter Ryd, Division of Cytology, Department of Pathology, Sahlgren's Hospital, Gothenburg, Sweden for letting us use illustrations of his case of desmoplastic small round cell tumour and Dr. Lennart Mellblom, Department of Pathology and Cytology, Kalmar Hospital, Kalmar, Sweden for contributing information regarding his case of ossifying fibromyxoid tumour. We also thank Prof. Frederik Mertens, Department of Clinical Genetics, University Hospital Lund, for providing figures 6 and 7.

Måns Åkerman
Henryk A. Domanski

I would like to thank Drs. Annika Dejmek and Karin Lindholm of the Department of Clinical Pathology and Cytology of the University Hospital MAS of Malmö, Sweden, for introducing me to the fantastic world of cytology and Dr. Måns Åkerman of the Department of Pathology and Cytology, University Hospital Lund, Sweden, my teacher and friend, for sharing his broad experience in aspiration cytology.

Henryk A. Domanski

Chapter 1

Soft Tissue Tumours – Basic Information

The incidence of soft tissue tumours is difficult to estimate, especially the ratio of benign to malignant. Benign lesions are usually estimated to be approximately 100 times more frequent than sarcomas. Sarcomas are relatively rare, constituting about 1% of all malignant tumours. In Sweden, the annual incidence of sarcomas of the locomotor system has been estimated to be 1.4/100,000. Age-specific incidence rates clearly demonstrate that soft tissue sarcomas of the locomotor system become more common with increasing age; in one study their incidence was 8.0/100,000 for patients 80 years or older.

Generally soft tissue sarcoma is more common in males but gender as well as age-related incidence depends on the histogenetic type.

Soft tissue tumours are usually classified histogenetically and within each group they are divided into benign lesions, sarcomas and intermediate or borderline tumours.

In this atlas, we use the classification proposed by Kempson et al. [1] and Weiss and Goldblum [2], respectively.

Since knowledge of the histotype of a sarcoma alone is not always sufficient to predict clinical course and choice of therapy, a number of grading systems, based on a variety of parameters, have been suggested and debated. The most frequent parameters used are cellularity, differentiation, cellular and nuclear pleomorphism, mitotic rate, necrosis and vascular invasion. The number of grades varies; two, three and four grades have been proposed. However, the histotype in itself may indicate tumour grade. For example, the extraskeletal Ewing's sarcoma (ES)/primitive neuroectodermal tumour (PNET) family of tumours, rhabdomyosarcoma and pleomorphic liposarcoma are all high-grade malignant, while well-differentiated liposarcoma, paucicellular myxoid liposarcoma, infantile fibrosarcoma and dermatofibrosarcoma protuberans are low grade. Provided that a FNA smear from a sarcoma is technically satisfactory and moderately cellular it is possible to grade most sarcomas into low-grade or high-grade categories.

The diagnostic workup of a soft tissue tumour before surgery includes site, type diagnosis and location in relation to the surrounding tissues, especially major nerves and vessels. Magnetic resonance imaging is usually best for this evaluation. For patients with sarcomas lung radiographs and sometimes computed tomography scans are obtained; it is important to determine whether metastatic disease is present in order to plan management.

In an attempt to predict outcome, to determine appropriate treatment and to make comparisons between the results of different centres, several staging systems have been proposed. However, there is no general consensus as to which one to use. Two which are commonly used are the American AJCC/UICC system (American Joint Committee/International Union Against Cancer) which is based on depth, grade and size, and the French FNCLCC system (French Federation of Cancer Centers) based on the same factors but with a more detailed definition of malignancy grade.

Chapter 2

Fine Needle Aspiration of Soft Tissue Tumours

Surgical Biopsy, Core Needle Biopsy or Fine Needle Aspiration in the Primary Diagnosis

In the majority of musculoskeletal tumour centres the definitive diagnosis of soft tissue tumours, especially suspected sarcomas, is based on the histopathological evaluation of a biopsy sample or a core needle biopsy with an outer diameter of 1.2–1.4 mm.

Although FNA with needles having an outer diameter of 0.4–0.8 mm has been a universally accepted diagnostic method in the definitive diagnosis of various tumour entities for many years, objections have been raised to FNA in the primary diagnosis of soft tissue tumours. The main objection has been the postulated inability to aspirate tumour material sufficient for reliable histotype diagnosis with a thin needle. Due to the numerous subtypes and morphological heterogeneity among specific entities, soft tissue tumours have been considered to pose some of the greatest diagnostic challenges in surgical pathology and routine light microscopy is often not sufficient for a diagnostic evaluation. Additional diagnostic methods such as histochemistry, immunohistochemistry, electron microscopy (EM), DNA ploidy analysis and chromosomal analysis and molecular genetics often have to be applied to reach a reliable diagnosis.

However, articles and book chapters on soft tissue tumours as a target for FNA began to appear at the beginning of the 1980s. The first case series published were often small and the diagnostic workup was not critically investigated.

In spite of a negative attitude to FNA among surgeons, oncologists and pathologists, it has been shown that the same advantages which have made FNA a first-choice diagnostic approach in breast tumours, thyroid tumours, salivary gland tumours or malignant lymphomas are also applicable in the diagnostic workup of a soft tissue tumour.

FNA of a suspected soft tissue tumour is an outpatient procedure. No anesthesia is necessary. One exception is the needling of soft tissue masses in children in whom a brief general anaesthesia may be needed. An evaluation of the aspirate within 10–15 min after needling is possible with a rapid haematoxylin-eosin (HE) or Diff-Quik stain. The adequacy of the material can thus be checked while the patient is waiting, and a preliminary diagnosis is sometimes possible. The purpose of a preliminary evaluation is 2-fold: it might give important information on the type of ancillary diagnostics that should be used and the surgeon can inform the patient and suggest further investigations or treatment at his/her first visit. Since the diagnosis and treatment of soft tissue sarcomas should preferably be centralized to multidisciplinary tumour centres, it is important as regards referred patients that the necessary information is obtained rapidly and the number of visits are as few as possible. Experience from the Musculoskeletal Tumour Centre at the University Hospital of Lund has shown that for patients referred to the centre for tumours suspicious of malignancy one visit was usually sufficient when the tumour proved to be benign at the combined evaluation of clinical examination, FNA diagnosis and radiographic examination, if any [3].

Core needle biopsy is also an outpatient procedure, but a preliminary diagnosis is less feasible than with FNA. FNA also permits sampling of different parts of large tumours to evaluate tumour heterogeneity, providing important information in, for example, lipomatous tumours.

A novel diagnostic approach, recently tested at our centre, is a combination of FNA and core needle biopsy in selected patients referred for FNA. The FNA as well as the core needle biopsy is performed by the cytologist at the same visit. This approach combines the advantages of both sampling methods: sampling from different parts of large tumours, a rapid preliminary report, the possibility to evaluate the tissue architecture in the core biopsy (often difficult in an FNA smear) (fig. 1a, b). In addition material sufficient for various ancillary methods such as immunohistochemistry, EM and cytogenetic/molecular genetic analyses [4] is obtained with greater certainty.

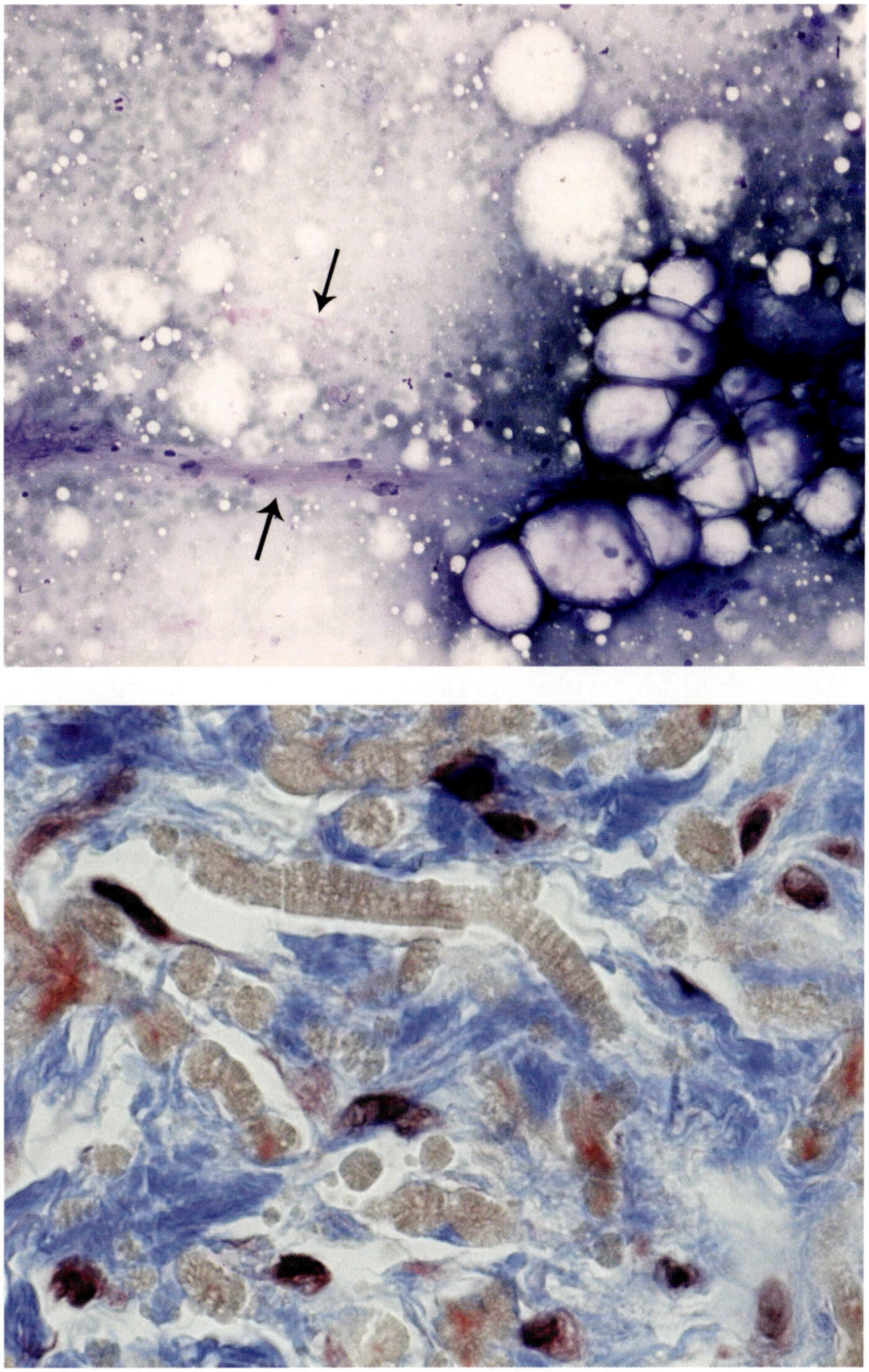

Fig. 1. The combined evaluation of FNA aspirates and core needle biopsy specimens may be necessary for a specific type-diagnosis of a soft tissue tumour. **a** FNA smear of an elastofibroma. Two fragments of elastic fibres are seen in the partly myxoid background (arrows). This material is not sufficient for a confident diagnosis. MGG. Medium magnification. **b** Core needle biopsy performed at the same session. The serrated degenerate elastic fibres can be easily seen. Masson's trichrome. Medium magnification.

Diagnostic Accuracy of Fine Needle Aspiration Biopsy

Several reports of diagnostic accuracy (i.e. differentiation of benign vs. malignant process) have been published. Accuracy has been greater than 90% in most publications but the case series have been small and the number of sarcomas evaluated often few [5–8]. Only a few large series from multidisplinary centres have been published. In a retrospective 20-year study of 517 tumours, 315 benign and 202 sarcoma cases of the extremities and trunk from the Musculoskeletal Tumour Centre, University Hospital of

Lund, there were 28 false diagnoses (5%), 14 false-negative and 14 false-positive. In 29 cases (6%) the material was insufficient for diagnosis (24/315 benign tumours and 5/202 sarcomas). An inconclusive diagnosis (uncertain whether benign or malignant) was given in 13 tumours (3%) while a correct diagnosis of benign tumour versus sarcoma was given for 447/475 tumours (94%) [9]. In this material the cytological malignancy grade (low/high) was assessed in 127/202 sarcomas and was correct in 103 (81%) and inconclusive in 24 (19%) [9].

In another study from the Musculoskeletal Tumour Centre at the Karolinska Hospital, Stockholm, comprising 342 tumours, the figures for accuracy were very similar [10].

Pitfalls in the Fine Needle Aspiration of Soft Tissue Tumours

There are three important limitations to FNA in the diagnosis of soft tissue tumours [11–12].

(1) The needle may miss the tumour and a false diagnosis is made on the basis of cells aspirated from the tissue surrounding it. Reactive cellular changes in the adipose tissue may mimick liposarcoma and pseudomalignant reactive changes in fibroblasts and myofibroblasts may suggest a pleomorphic sarcoma. This diagnostic difficulty most often occurs when small, deep-seated, inter- or intramuscular tumours are needled. It is important that the person performing the aspiration has enough experience to be able to evaluate whether the material obtained might be consistent with the tumour in question (age, history, site, size, and palpatory findings). It is recommended that small, deep-seated tumours be needled with ultrasound guidance.

(2) Insufficient or technically suboptimal material may result in a false diagnosis or preclude any diagnosis at all. The temptation of making a diagnosis on quantitatively or qualitatively insufficient material must be resisted. It is a fact that some tumours are difficult to diagnose by FNA. Vascular tumours most often yield predominantly blood and very few cells and in various tumours rich in dilated vessels the aspirates may be very bloody but contain very few tumour cells. Another difficulty is to obtain a sufficient number of cells from tumours with an abundant collagenous or hyalinized background matrix. Extensive necrosis, cystic degeneration or haemorrhage can also make diagnostic aspiration very difficult. In general, however, with adequate sampling, it is possible to obtain sufficient material for diagnosis.

(3) Misinterpretation of the material is, however, the main cause of false diagnoses. There are a number of well-documented diagnostic difficulties, which shall be discussed in the following chapters. Besides misinterpretation of the material there is yet another cause for a false diagnosis. In the case of rare tumours or so-called 'new entities', cytological criteria which permit accurate evaluation may not have been established. Comparative histological-cytological studies of reasonably large series are often lacking. Examples of rare tumours and new entities, hitherto difficult to diagnose correctly as benign or malignant, as well as to type, are chondroid lipoma, perineurioma, aggressive angiomyxoma, solitary fibrous tumour of soft tissue, mixed tumour of soft tissue, parachordoma and spindle cell liposarcoma.

Complications of Fine Needle Aspiration of Soft Tissue Tumours

In our experience of FNA of more than 25 years in the primary diagnosis of soft tissue tumours in patients referred to our Musculoskeletal Tumour Centre we have never experienced any severe complication. Patients have, at most, complained of tenderness and, in cases of subcutaneous tumours, of haemorrhage. We have not seen a single case of infection and never experienced clinical signs of sarcoma cell seeding in the needle track. It is to be remembered that FNA is the least tissue-destructive invasive diagnostic method.

Fine Needle Aspiration Cytology Procedure

Practical Considerations

The aspiration technique is the same as for other targets for FNA. We have found that a syringe holder which allows aspiration with one hand is essential for success. Needles wider than 22 gauge (0.7 mm) are very rarely necessary. The length of the needle depends on the site of the tumour. For deep-seated tumours, needles with a stylet are recommended. The stylet strengthens the needle and prevents cells from surrounding tissues from being included in the smears. Thorough palpation and estimation of size, site and consistency of the tumour is essential. Since the surgeon often may want to determine the point of insertion of the needle, close communication with the surgeon is mandatory. If the surgeon does not indicate the insertion point, the tumour is needled through the vertex. In case of suspected sarcoma the insertion point can, at the request of the surgeon, be tattooed so that the needle track can be removed at surgery (fig. 2). Our policy is to perform at most 5 FNA passes, all through

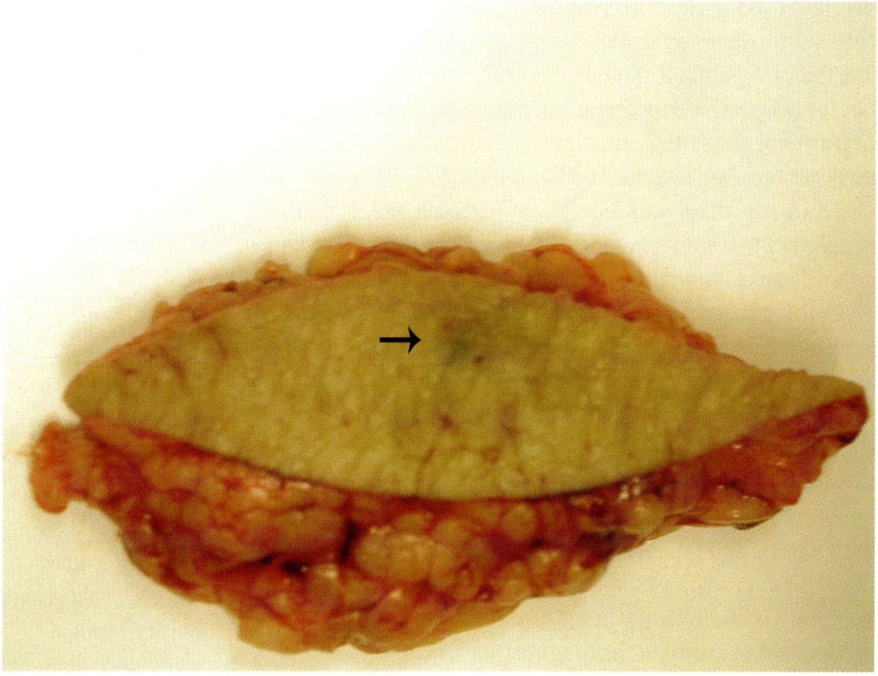

Fig. 2. A subcutaneous sarcoma removed with the overlying skin. The insertion point is marked by the tattoo (arrow).

the same insertion point. Due to tumour tissue heterogeneity, especially in large tumours, it is important to sample tissue from different parts of the tumour.

The microscopic evaluation should be based on both wet-fixed [HE or Papanicolaou (Pap)] and air-dried [May-Grünwald-Giemsa (MGG) or Diff-Quik] smears.

The wet-fixed material is superior for evaluation of nuclear details such as chromatin structure and nucleoli while the MGG staining gives excellent information on cytoplasmic details and the background matrix.

Cytodiagnosis

One common objection to FNA in the primary diagnosis of soft tissue tumours is the supposed inability to correctly and reliably diagnose the numerous different histotypes in smears. However, the necessary diagnostic level for a soft tissue tumour is determined by the primary treatment envisaged in the individual case. First of all the surgeon must know whether the tumour in question is a true soft tissue lesion/tumour or a soft tissue metastasis or a primary soft tissue lymphoma. In case of sarcoma the standard treatment in the majority of cases is primary radical surgery, sometimes followed by radiotherapy. The type of surgical intervention depends more on the site (subcutaneous or deep), size and the relation of the sarcoma to vessels, nerve bundles and periosteum than on the histotype. Thus a reliable diagnosis of sarcoma is sufficient for the surgeon in those cases where primary radical surgery is the proposed treatment.

When the treatment includes neoadjuvant therapy (radiotherapy or chemotherapy) followed by surgery, the FNA diagnosis must equal that of a histopathological evaluation as regards histotype and malignancy grade.

At present neoadjuvant therapy is used for rhabdomyosarcoma, neuroblastoma, the extraskeletal Ewing/PNET family of tumours and in some centres selected cases of soft tissue sarcomas.

On the other hand, in case of a benign soft tissue tumour or reactive soft tissue lesion the surgeon often wants to know the histotype in order to inform the patient of the two treatment options: observation/follow-up or local excision. Observation may be suggested in the pseudosarcomatous soft tissue lesions, especially nodular fasciitis and pseudomalignant myositis ossificans, and in case of lipoma or neurilemoma and desmoid fibromatosis. A shelling out of the tumour is sufficient treatment for most benign soft tissue tumours except desmoid fibromatosis, which requires more extensive margins due to its infiltrative growth.

Classification of the Cytodiagnosis

Standardized reporting is an advantage both to the surgeon and to the cytopathologist. At our Musculoskeletal Tumour Centre we have for many years used four main diagnoses: benign, sarcoma, other malignancy or inconclusive. Inconclusive means either that the material is insufficent for diagnosis (poor yield, necrosis, cystic degeneration or technically unsatisfactory) or that it is not possible to reliably decide whether a malignant tumour is a true soft tissue sarcoma or not, or whether a soft tissue tumour is benign or malignant. In our experience the term 'inconclusive diagnosis' is better than various expressions of uncertainty [57].

The main diagnoses benign or sarcoma are, if possible, supplemented with a suggested histotype diagnosis and in case of sarcoma, malignancy grade (low or high).

Cytological criteria for specific histotype diagnoses have been evaluated in comparative studies of series of FNA smears and histopathological sections from well-defined histotypes, and cytological criteria for a specific-type diagnosis have been suggested and published in a number of tumour types, benign as well as sarcoma (table 1). The cytological findings in many uncommon tumours and 'new' entities are mainly described in case reports and reliable diagnostic criteria are at present lacking. However, it is possible to give a confident diagnosis of benignity or malignancy in most of these cases.

In order to faciliate the diagnostic workup of a soft tissue tumour FNA sample, smears may be classified according to the principal microscopic pattern. Although there is a certain overlap between patterns, such a categorization may be useful in the endeavour to reach a confident diagnosis of benignity or malignancy, to suggest a type-specific diagnosis as well as in the recognition of important differential diagnoses. This approach is recommended in particular to cytopathologists working in a general institution not related to a specialized orthopaedic oncology unit as a basis for appropriate referral to such a unit.

In chapter 4 we propose a classification of this type of FNA samples from soft tissue tumours.

Table 1. Benign soft tissue tumours/lesions and sarcomas

	References
Tumour/lesion	
Nodular fasciitis	13
Proliferative myositis and fasciitis	14
Pseudomalignant myositis ossificans	15
Lipomatous tumours, benign	16–19
Neurilemoma	20–22
Granular cell tumour	23
Intramuscular myxoma	24
Angioleiomyoma	25
Sarcoma	
MFH	26, 27
Myxofibrosarcoma	28, 29
Leiomyosarcoma	30
Liposarcoma	16, 17, 31, 32
MPNST	33, 34
Synovial sarcoma	35–38
Rhabdomyosarcoma	39–44
Neuroblastoma	45, 46
Angiosarcoma	47–49
Alveolar soft part sarcoma	50, 51
Clear cell sarcoma	52
Dermatofibrosarcoma protuberans	53, 54
Epithelioid sarcoma	55, 56

Suggested diagnostic criteria for a specific diagnosis based on comparative histological and cytological studies.

The Final Evaluation of a Soft Tissue Tumour Aspirate

Experience has taught us that the diagnosis and treatment should be based on the combined evaluation of clinical data, radiographic investigations and cytodiagnosis, the same concept of triple diagnosis that has been the consensus for breast lesions for many years (clinical data, mammography and cytodiagnosis) [57, 58]. The optimal workup is to discuss this combined information for each patient in a multidisciplinary team of a musculoskeletal tumour centre. The team decides whether available data, including the cytodiagnosis, are sufficient for definitive treatment. Generally an inconclusive cytodiagnosis or a cytodiagnosis not consistent with clinical or radiographic data leads to a repeat aspiration or a core or open biopsy. If mutilating surgery is considered a biopsy is performed unless the cytodiagnosis is as certain as a histopathological evaluation. In the re-evaluation of our 20-year material about 5% of the sarcoma cases underwent open biopsy and in 1 out of 202 sarcomas the triple diagnosis failed [9].

Ancillary Diagnostic Methods Supplementing the Cytodiagnosis

The use of special diagnostic methods is often necessary to correctly assess a soft tissue tumour. The same methods used in histopathology are applicable to FNA aspirates.

In spite of the widespread use of immunohistochemistry in the diagnosis of soft tissue tumours the value of immunocytochemistry (IC) as a diagnostic aid has not yet been evaluated in large series. Published case reports and our own experience have, however, indicated that IC is a valuable asset in the differential diagnosis between pleomorphic sarcoma and soft tissue metastases from anaplastic carcinoma or melanoma, and between pleomorphic sarcoma and the primary soft tissue presentation of anaplastic large cell lymphoma (ALCL). We have also found IC helpful in the differential diagnosis of various spindle cell tumours such as

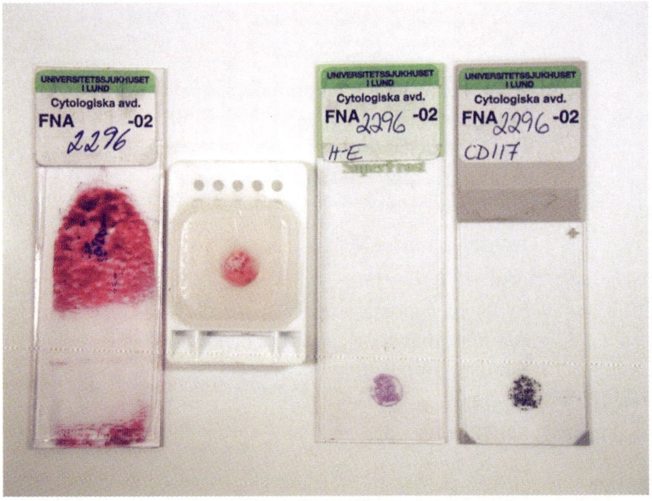

a

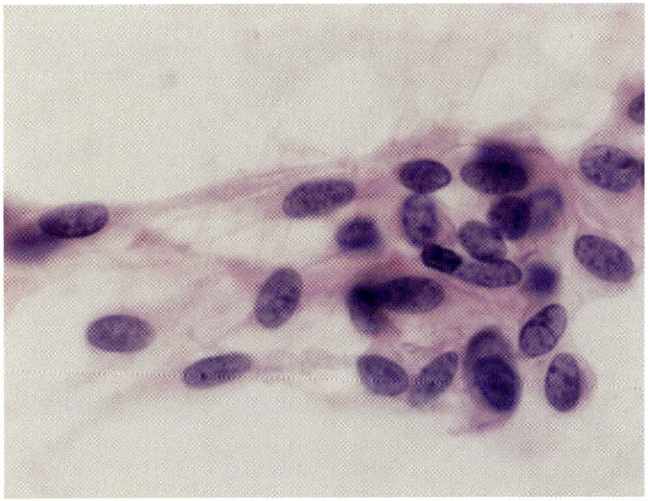

b

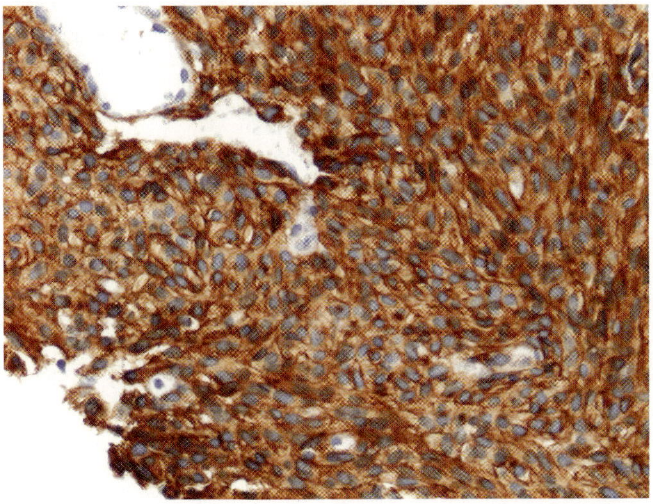

c

Fig. 3. The combined evaluation of routinely stained smears and immunohistochemical staining of a cell block 'microbiopsy' is often sufficient for a specific type-diagnosis. **a** Cytology slide and the cell block 'microbiopsy'. **b** In this particular case a suspected GIST metastasis was needled. The routinely stained smear shows part of a spindle cell sarcoma. HE. High magnification. **c** Positive staining with CD117, section from the cell block.

Table 2. Useful antibodies in the diagnosis of soft tissue sarcoma and other malignancies

	Tumour
Antibody[1]	
Muscle-specific actin	Leiomyosarcoma ~80–90%+
	Rhabdomyosarcoma ~90%+
Smooth muscle actin (SMA)	Leiomyosarcoma ~90%+
Desmin	Leiomyosarcoma ~70–75%+
	Rhabdomyosarcoma ~90–95%+
	DSRCT ~90%+
	Extrarenal malignant rhabdoid tumour (some)
Caldesmon	Leiomyosarcoma
Myoglobin	Rhabdomyosarcoma ~40%+
MyoD1	Rhabdomyosarcoma >90%+
S-100 protein	MPNST ~40–50%+
	Round cell liposarcoma ~60–70%+
	Clear cell sarcoma ~80%+
	EMC ~20–40%+
	Synovial sarcoma ~30%+

Table 2 (continued)

	Tumour
CD34	Dermatofibrosarcoma protuberans ~90–95%+ Malignant haemangiopericytoma ~50%+ Epithelioid sarcoma ~50%+ Angiosarcoma ~60–80%+ GIST ~80%+
CD31	Angiosarcoma ~90%+
CD99	ES/PNET ~>95%+ Synovial sarcoma ~60%+ Alveolar rhabdomyosarcoma (some) Solitary fibrous tumour
Neuron-specific enolase (NSE)	Neuroblastoma PNET DSRCT
Chromogranin	Neuroblastoma (often in undifferentiated tumours) PNET
Synaptophysin	Neuroblastoma (often in undifferentiated tumours) PNET
Cytokeratin	Synovial sarcoma ~50–90%+ Epithelioid sarcoma ~90%+ Angiosarcoma (epithelioid angiosarcoma often +) Leiomyosarcoma ~30%+ DSRCT >90%+ Extrarenal malignant rhabdoid tumour
EMA	Synovial sarcoma ~50–95%+ Epithelioid sarcoma Epithelioid angiosarcoma
CD117 (c-kit)	GIST (almost all)
Antibody[2]	
Cytokeratin	Carcinoma
EMA	Carcinoma Anaplastic large cell lymphoma
CD30	Hodgkin's lymphoma Anaplastic large cell lymphoma
CD3, CD79a, CD10, Tdt	Lymphoblastic lymphoma
CD45, CD3, CD20	Non-Hodgkin's lymphoma in general
Alk1	Anaplastic large cell lymphoma
CD138	Plasmacytoma
MPO	Granulocytic sarcoma (myelosarcoma)
HMB45, Melan A	Malignant melanoma

1 Useful in the diagnosis of soft tissue sarcoma.
2 Useful in the differential diagnosis of other malignancies.

neurilemoma, leiomyosarcoma, solitary fibrous tumour and occasionally in the type diagnosis of synovial sarcoma. IC is an important diagnostic asset in the specific diagnosis of angiosarcoma and small round cell sarcomas.

We have found IC on cell block preparations from aspirates more reliable than on cytocentrifuge preparations. All antibodies used in soft tissue tumour diagnosis are suitable for formalin-fixed and paraffin-embedded tissue and well suited for the small tissue of successful cell block preparations (fig. 3a–c) (table 2).

The diagnostic value of EM is still significant in spite of the vast use of immunostaining. EM in the diagnostic

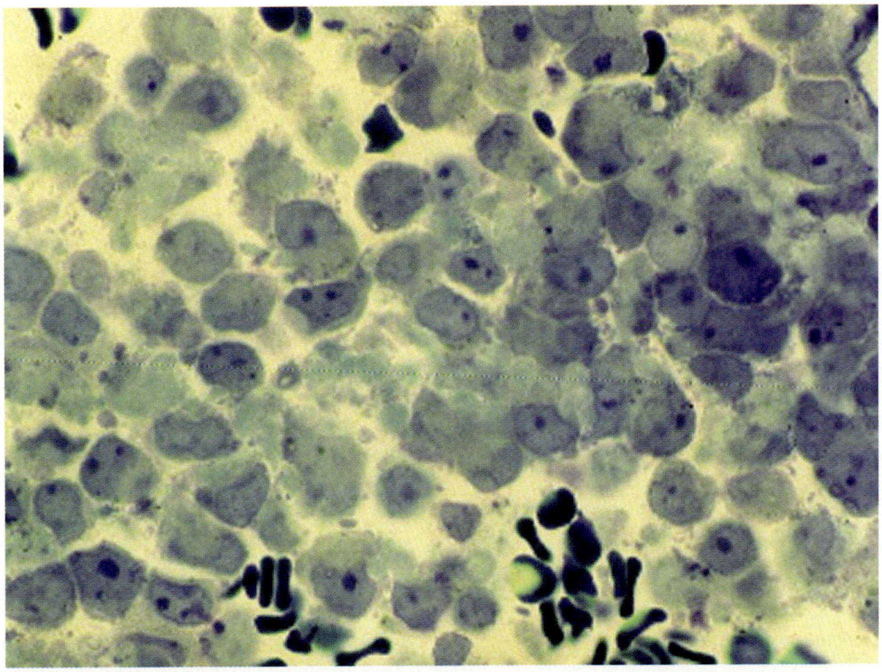

a

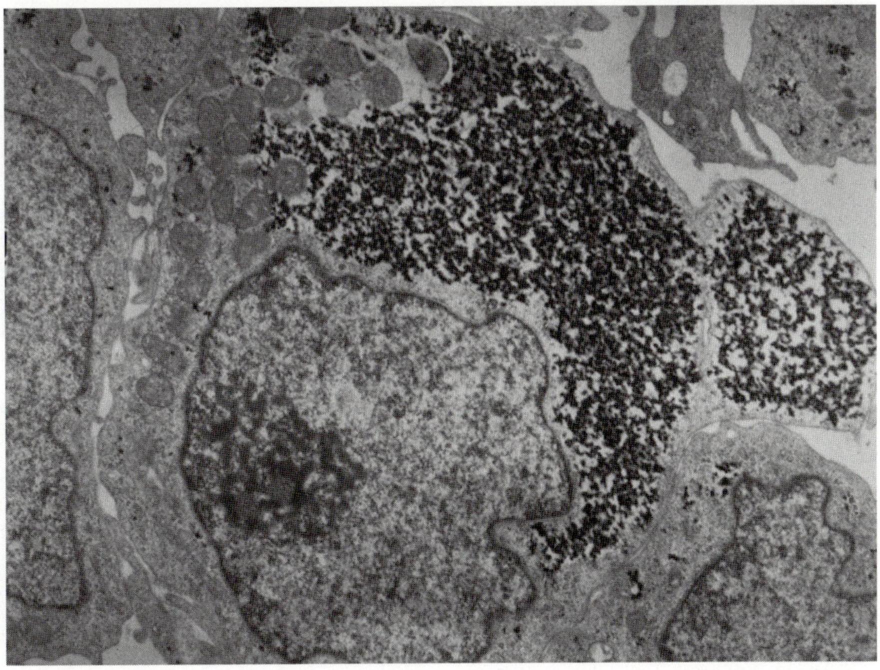

b

Fig. 4. FNA sample processed for EM. **a** The microbiopsy from which the cells to be examined are chosen. **b** Electron micrograph of the prepared specimen. In this case a conventional ES. The abundant cytoplasmic glycogen is easily seen.

evaluation of FNA aspirates has been thoroughly investigated [60, 61]. We and others have found EM especially valuable in the classification of small round cell sarcomas (fig. 4a, b), in the differential diagnosis of various spindle cell tumours and in selected soft tissue tumours which exhibit specific ultrastructural features such as premelanosomes in clear cell sarcoma or Weibel-Palade bodies in vascular tumours.

Flow-cytometric as well as image-cytometric DNA ploidy analyses (FCM and ICM, respectively) have been performed on several series of soft tissue sarcomas, mixed histotypes as well as specific entities. Although an unequivocal non-diploid cell population strongly favours a high-grade sarcoma (fig. 5), DNA ploidy analysis has proved to be of limited value in the diagnosis and prognostication of soft tissue sarcoma. A number of high-grade sarcomas may display a diploid cell population.

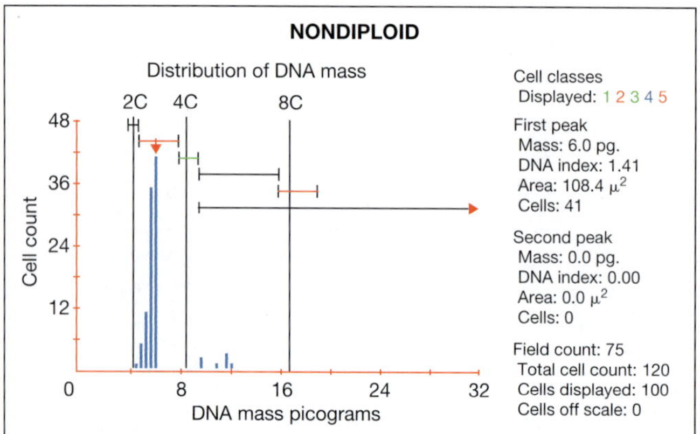

Area	Min.	Max.	Modal D.I.	Mean D.I.	S.D.	C.V.	%Cells	# Cells	Description
A	0.92	1.11	1.09	1.09	0.00	0.00	0.83	1	
B	1.11	1.84	1.39	1.35	0.07	5.21	76.67	92	
C	1.84	2.22	0.00	0.00	0.00	0.00	0.00	0	
D	2.22	3.68	2.72	2.58	0.22	8.37	5.83	7	
E	3.68	4.44	0.00	0.00	0.00	0.00	0.00	0	
F	2.22	17.81	2.72	2.58	0.22	8.37	5.83	7	

Fig. 5. Image cytometry of a high-grade malignant soft tissue sarcoma. Aneuploid cell population.

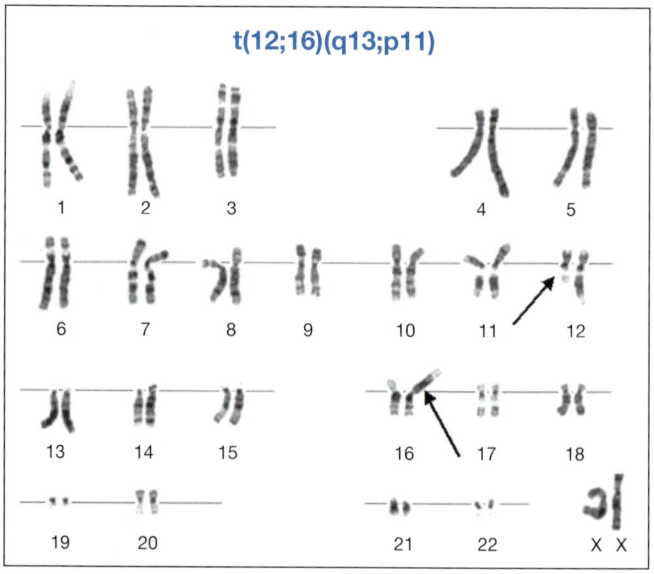

Fig. 6. FNA of a myxoid liposarcoma processed for karyotyping. The typical translocation t(12;16) is marked.

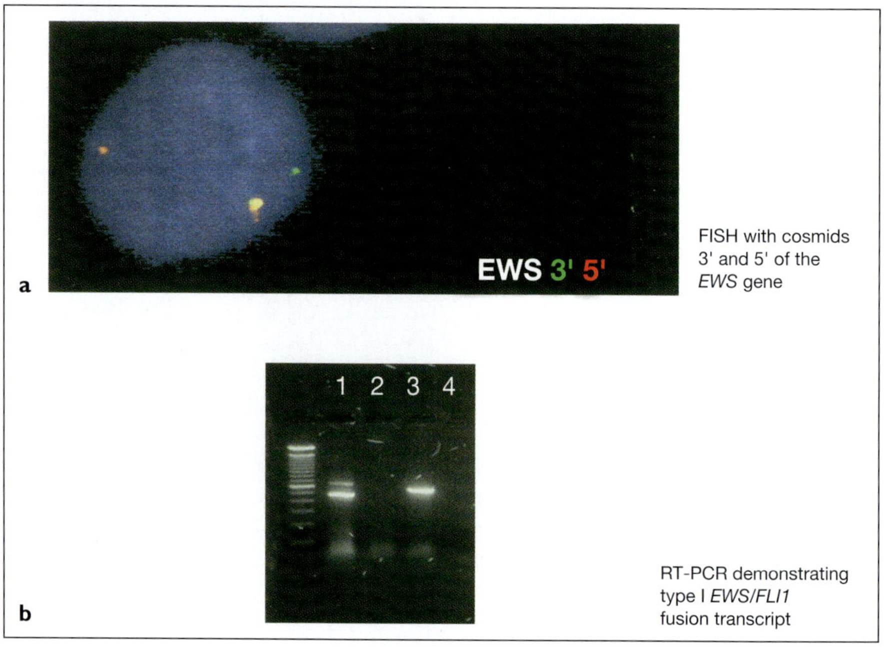

Fig. 7. a FISH prepared from an air-dried unstained smear of a tumour of the ES/PNET family. **b** RT-PCR of the same case. 1 = Patient; 2 = negative control; 3 = positive control; 4 = blank.

FCM as well as ICM can be performed on fine needle aspirates. One advantage with ICM is that previously stained aspirates may be destained, restained with Feulgen and analyzed. We have found DNA ploidy analysis of limited diagnostic value in the evaluation of a soft tissue tumour aspirate in the differential diagnosis of benignity and malignancy. An unequivocal non-diploid cell population indicates sarcoma and furthermore a high-grade sarcoma [45] while a diploid or tetraploid histogram is of no diagnostic value. A disadvantage with FCM is that false diploid histograms may occur [62, 63]. Through comparative FCM and ICM analyses on the same tissue specimen it has become evident

Table 3. Chromosomal aberrations in soft tissue sarcoma

Sarcoma	Chromosomal aberration	Genes involved	Performed on FNA (Ref. No.)
ES/PNET	t(11;22)(q24;q12)	*FLI1-EWS*	64, 66
Alveolar rhabdomyosarcoma	t(2;13)(q35;q14)	*PAX3-FKHR*	67
DSRCT	t((11;22)(p13;q12)	*WT1-EWS*	127
Synovial sarcoma	t(X;18)(p11.2;q11.2)	*SSX1-SYT* *SSX''-SYT*	65
Clear cell sarcoma	t(12;22)(q13;q12)	*AFT1-EWS*	
EMC	t(9;22)(q22;q12)	*TEC-EWS*	68

that diploid or inconclusive FCM histograms in tissue specimens as well as in aspirates should be supplemented with ICM to avoid false results.

Cytogenetic analysis has emerged as a promising diagnostic adjunct in soft tissue tumour diagnosis. Karyotyping, fluorescent in situ hybridization (FISH) and molecular genetic analysis can be performed on FNA from musculoskeletal tumours [64–68] (fig. 6). FISH or reverse transcriptase-polymerase chain reaction (RT-PCR; when the genes involved in a diagnostic chromosomal aberration, most often a translocation, are known) are easier to perform on FNA, because the number of cells necessary for these analyses are far less than for conventional karyotyping, and dividing cells are not necessary (fig. 7). The hitherto known diagnostic chromosomal aberrations are listed in table 3.

Chapter 3

The Cytology of Benign, Pseudomalignant Reactive Changes in Fibrous Tissue, Adipose Tissue and Striated Muscle in Fine Needle Aspiration Samples

One reason for a false-positive diagnosis of sarcoma in a soft tissue tumour aspirate is the misinterpretation of benign, reactive cellular changes in benign conditions.

Fibrous Tissue

Normal fibroblasts/myofibroblasts appear in FNA samples as spindle-shaped cells with slender cytoplasm, often with elongated cytoplasmic processes. The nuclei are rounded, ovoid or fusiform with regular chromatin and small nucleoli, if any. The cells are seen either as dissociated or in small clusters or runs of loosely attached cells. Stripped nuclei are not uncommon (fig. 8).

Reactive fibroblasts/myofibroblasts show, irrespective of cause, a wide variation in size and shape. The cells become polyhedral or triangular, often with rather abundant cytoplasm. They may show angulated cytoplasmic extensions or cytoplasmic

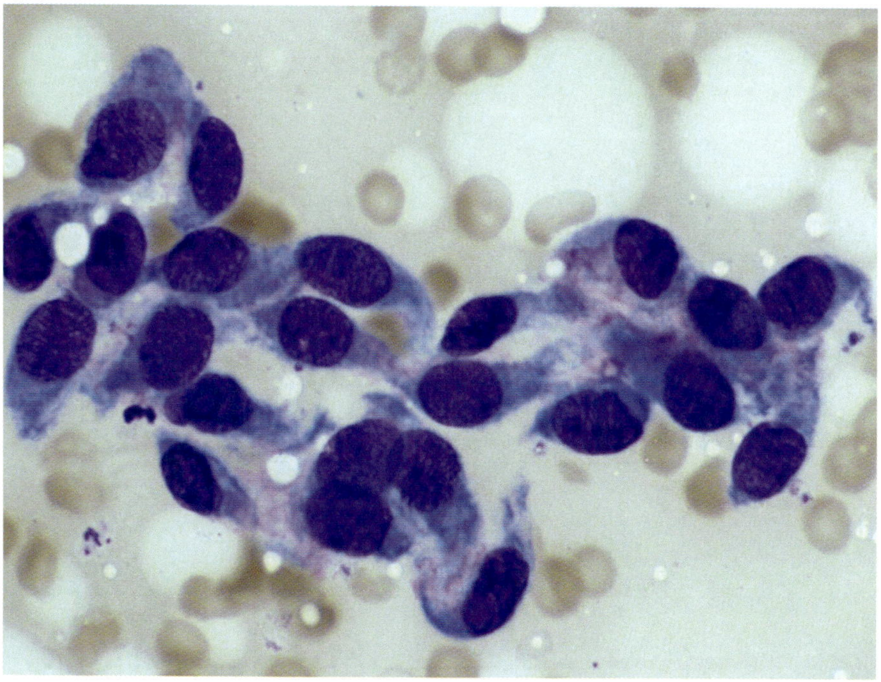

Fig. 8. Normal fibroblasts in an FNA biopsy. A run of loosely cohesive cells with ovoid, uniform nuclei, regular chromatin and bipolar cytoplasm. MGG. Medium magnification.

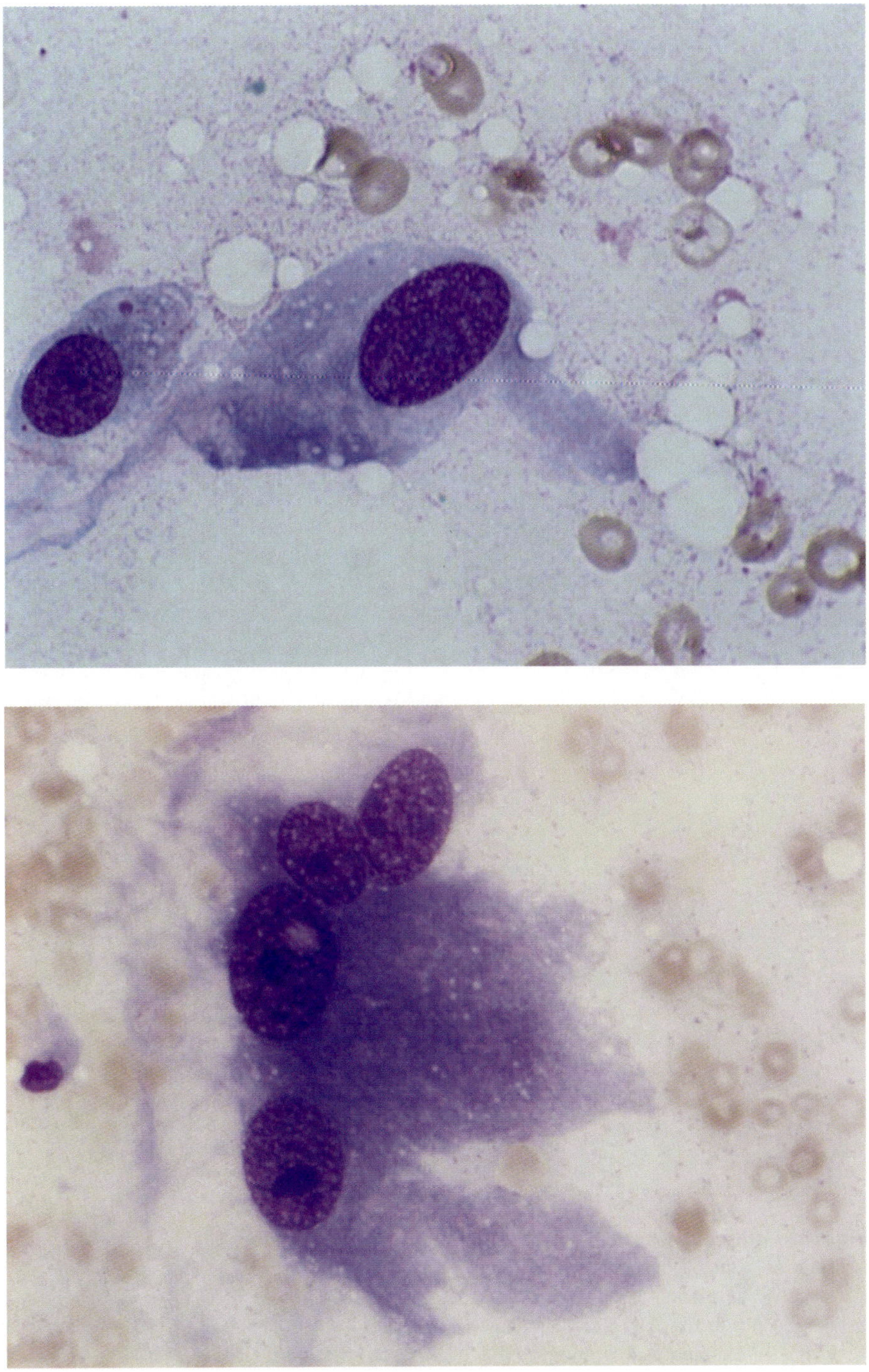

a

b

Fig. 9. Example of reactive fibroblast/myofibroblast. **a** Larger than normal fibroblasts with more abundant cytoplasm with angulated extensions and large nuclei with prominent nucleoli. **b** A multinucleated, ganglioncell-like reactive fibroblast. MGG. High magnification.

processes. The nuclei vary in size and shape (rounded, ovoid, spindle-shaped) and nucleoli may be large and prominent. Binucleated cells are not uncommon (fig. 9a, b).

Typical examples of the pleomorphic appearance of reactive fibroblasts/myofibroblasts are seen in the pseudomalignant, benign soft tissue lesions, especially in nodular fasciitis and proliferative myositis.

Adipose Tissue

Normal adipose tissue is seen as small fragments or clusters of large cells with abundant univacuolated cytoplasm and small, dark, regular nuclei. A discrete network of thin capillaries is often observed. Dissociated adipocytes are uncommon.

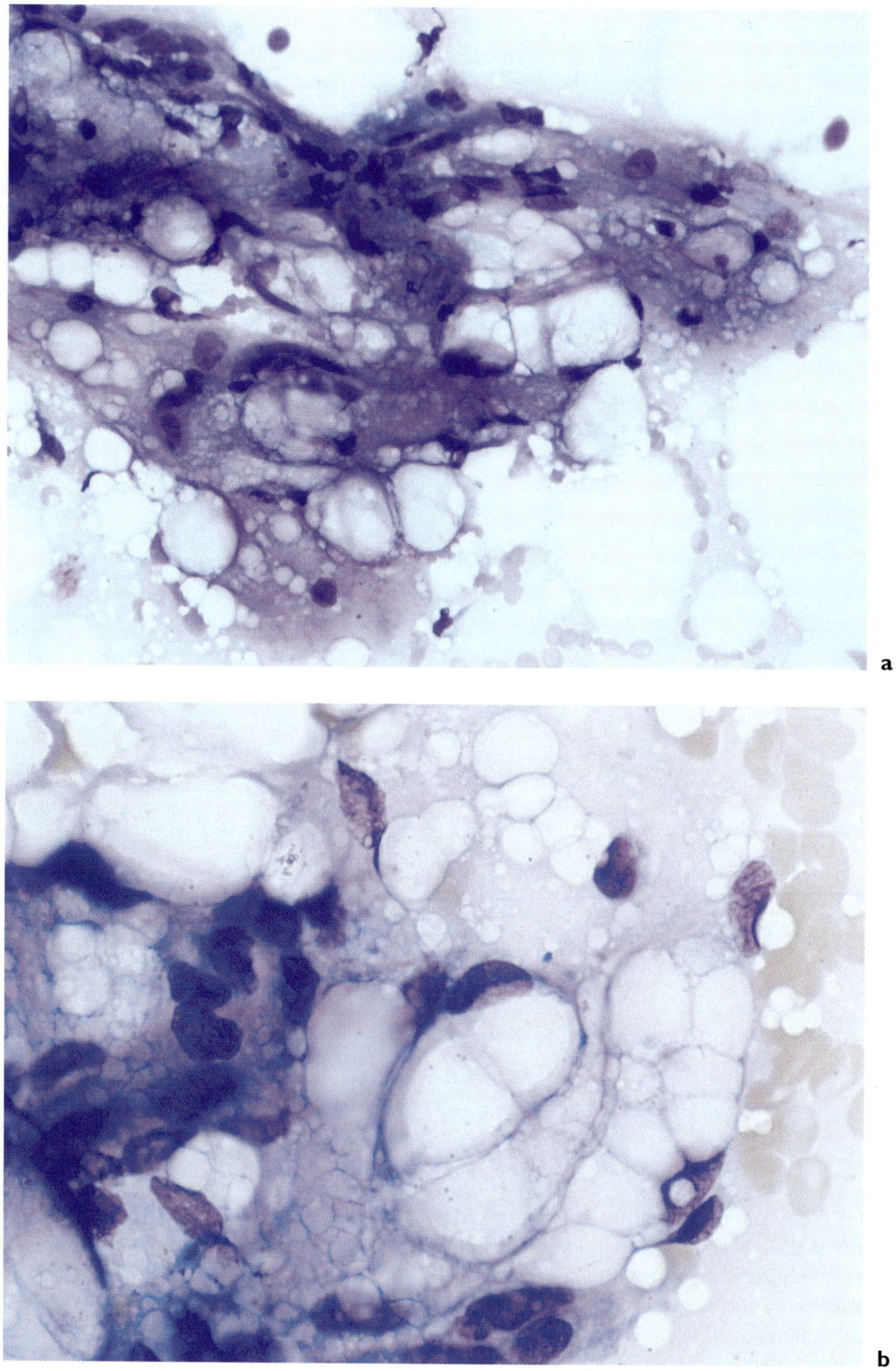

Fig. 10. Cellular changes in adipose tissue. **a** Partly myxoid background and different-sized adipocytes. **b** Increased cellularity due to the presence of fibroblasts and histiocytes. **a**, **b** MGG. Medium magnification.

In reactive states, posttraumatic, inflammatory or in adipose tissue bordering various tumours, the adipose tissue may exhibit a myxoid-like background, the capillary network is more pronounced, the adipocytes vary in size and the fat fragments appear more cellular than normal due to the presence of fibroblasts and histiocytes (fig. 10a, b). Histiocytes with foamy or vacuolated cytoplasm appear between the fat fragments.

Striated Muscle

Normal striated muscle in FNA samples is seen as fragments of muscle fibres with small dark nuclei and a more or less evident striation. The fibres are densely eosinophilic in HE and dark blue in MGG. Regenerating muscle fibres appear in FNA samples as multinucleated cells of varying

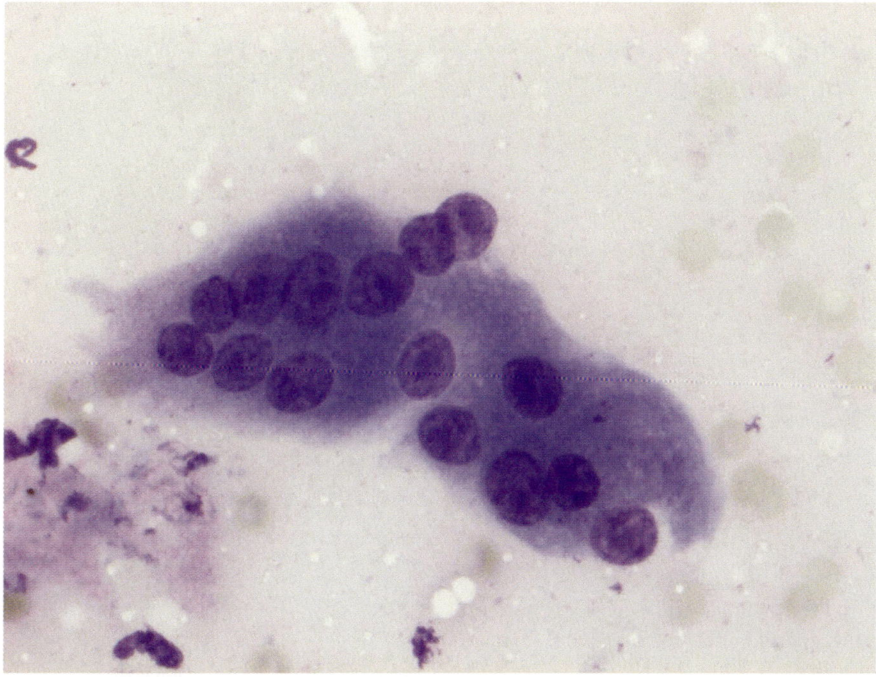

11a

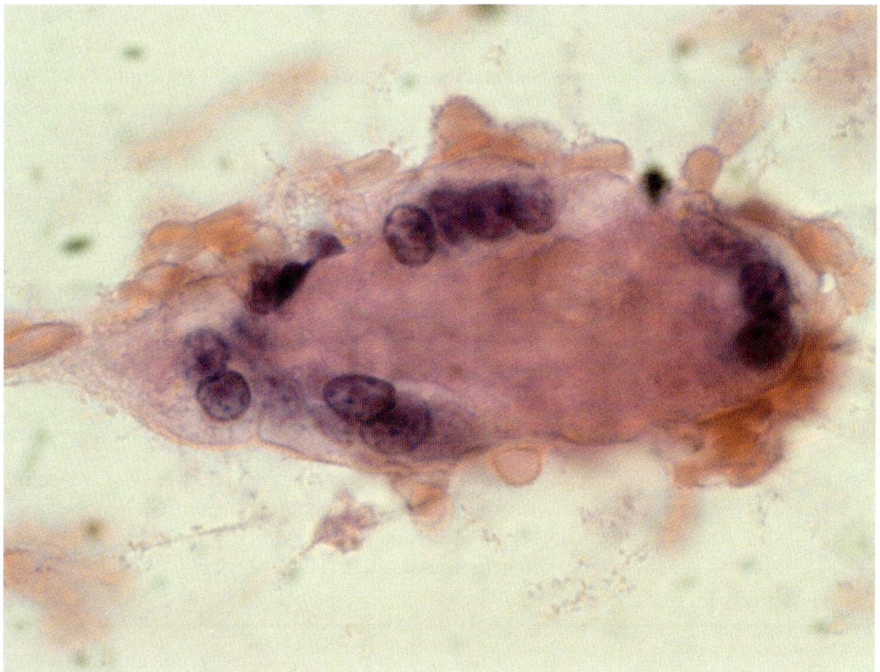

11b

Fig. 11. Examples of regenerating striated muscle fibres. **a** Typical 'muscle giant cells' with rows of nuclei and dark blue cytoplasm. MGG. High magnification. **b** The cytoplasm is eosinophilic in HE. High magnification.

size and shape. They are rounded, polyhedral, strap-shaped or tadpole-like. The cytoplasm is densely eosinophilic in HE and dark blue in MGG. The multiple nuclei are moderately large, uniform in size and often harbour a prominent nucleolus. The nuclei are typically arranged in rows, eccentrically located (fig. 11a–c).

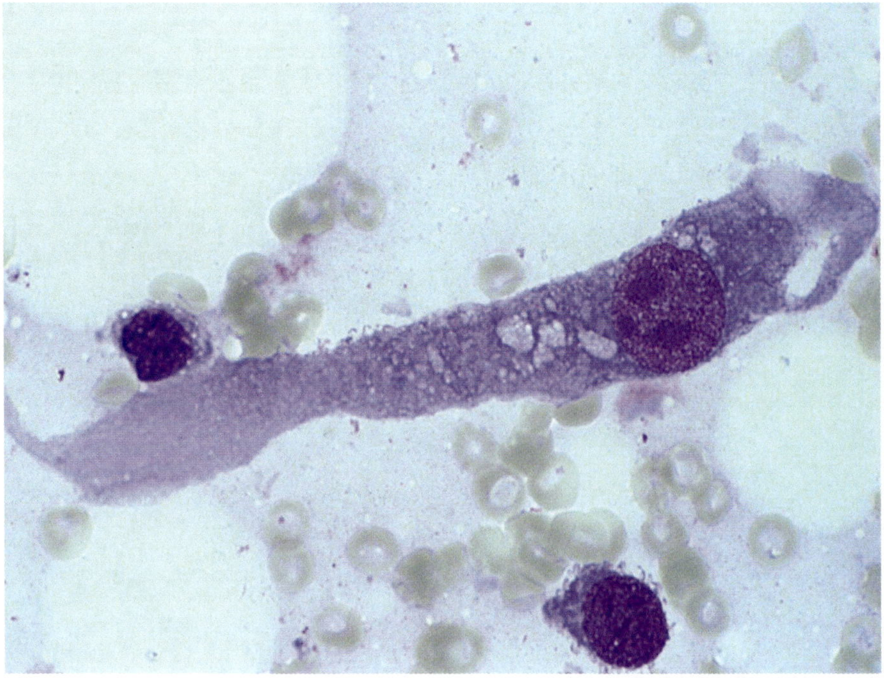

11c

Fig. 11c. A uninuclear, tadpole-like regenerating striated muscle fibre. MGG. High magnification.

Table 4. A summary of benign 'pseudomalignant changes' in aspirated material from fibrous and adipose tissue and striated muscle

Tissue	Cellular changes	Lesions
Fibroblasts/myofibroblasts	Variation in size, variation in shape; elongated, triangular, polygonal, plump with cytoplasmic extensions; variable nuclear shape and size; binucleation; prominent nucleoli	Benign pseudosarcomatous soft tissue lesions Posttraumatic states
Adipose tissue	Increased vascularity; increased cellularity (fibroblasts, endothelial cells, histiocytes); multivacuolated cytoplasm in adipocytes; uni- or multinucleated histocytes between fat fragments (lipophages)	Status after fat necrosis Posttraumatic states Adipose tissue surrounding various non-adipose tumours
Striated muscle	Multi- or uninucleated regenerating muscle fibres ('muscle giant cells'); occasionally presence of tadpole-like regenerating muscle fibres; prominent; nucleoli; dense eosinophilic (HE) or dark blue (MGG) cytoplasm	Aspirates from tumours/lesions infiltrating striated muscle Examples: intramuscular lipoma, intramuscular myxoma, desmoid, fibromatosis colli

Regenerating muscle fibres are mainly found within FNA samples from tumours infiltrating striated muscle. Typical examples are infantile fibromatosis colli and desmoid fibromatosis.

A summary of the reactive cytological changes in fibrous tissue, adipose tissue and striated muscle is presented in table 4.

Chapter 4

The Cytological Features of Soft Tissue Tumours in Fine Needle Aspiration Smears Classified According to Histotype

Adipocytic Tumours

Adipocytic tumours are the most common soft tissue tumours due to the common subcutaneous lipoma. Furthermore liposarcoma is one of the most frequent soft tissue sarcomas. The diagnosis of adipocytic tumours by FNA is predominantly based on the examination of routinely stained smears, as is the case with the histopathological diagnosis. IC is a useful adjunct in some of the lipoma variants. Cytogenetic analysis, however, is gaining importance as a diagnostic asset in the evaluation, and most probably FISH analysis of FNA smears will be of value in the type-specific diagnosis of lipomatous tumours in the future. Relatively type-specific chromosomal aberrations in adipocytic tumours are listed in table 6.

Subcutaneous lipoma is a common target for FNA, intramuscular lipoma is relatively common while lipoma variants such as angiolipoma, spindle cell and pleomorphic lipoma, hibernoma, and lipoblastoma are infrequently needled. Chondroid lipoma as well as myelolipoma are, due to their rarity, only occasionally the target for FNA.

Benign Adipocytic Tumours

Subcutaneous Lipoma

The proximal extremities and the trunk are the most common sites. Size is variable but seldom exceeds 10 cm. Subcutaneous lipoma is uncommon in children but does occur.

Histopathology

Subcutaneous lipomas have a lobular pattern and are composed of mature fat cells, which vary slightly in shape and size. The nuclei are small and uniform. The microscopic appearance is very much like that of normal subcutaneous fat.

Subcutaneous lipomas are well vascularized.

Fibrous connective tissue is occasionally admixed with the lipoma tissue, in which case the lesion is classified as fibrolipoma. Subcutaneous lipoma may also be partly myxoid (myxolipoma) or exhibit cartilaginous metaplasia (chondrolipoma).

Secondary changes such as focal fat necrosis may also occur with the presence of clusters or strands of macrophages with foamy or vacuolated cytoplasm (lipophages).

Cytological features of subcutaneous lipoma (fig. 12a, b)

Adipose tissue fragments of variable size
Few dissociated adipocytes
Fragments composed of large univacuolated mature adipocytes with eccentric small dark, uniform nuclei
Capillary strands present in the adipose tissue fragments

Differential diagnosis

Normal subcutaneous adipose tissue
Chondroid lipoma
Well-differentiated liposarcoma (atypical lipomatous tumour)
Myxoid liposarcoma

Comments

As aspirates from subcutaneous lipoma have principally the same appearance in FNA smears as normal subcutaneous adipose tissue it is important to certify that the needle has been placed within the lipoma.

Many subcutaneous lipomas exhibit reactive cellular changes such as increased vascularity, scattered or clustered adipocytes with multivacuolated cytoplasm and histiocytes with foamy cytoplasm (lipophages) between fragments. These reactive changes may suggest a well-differentiated liposarcoma.

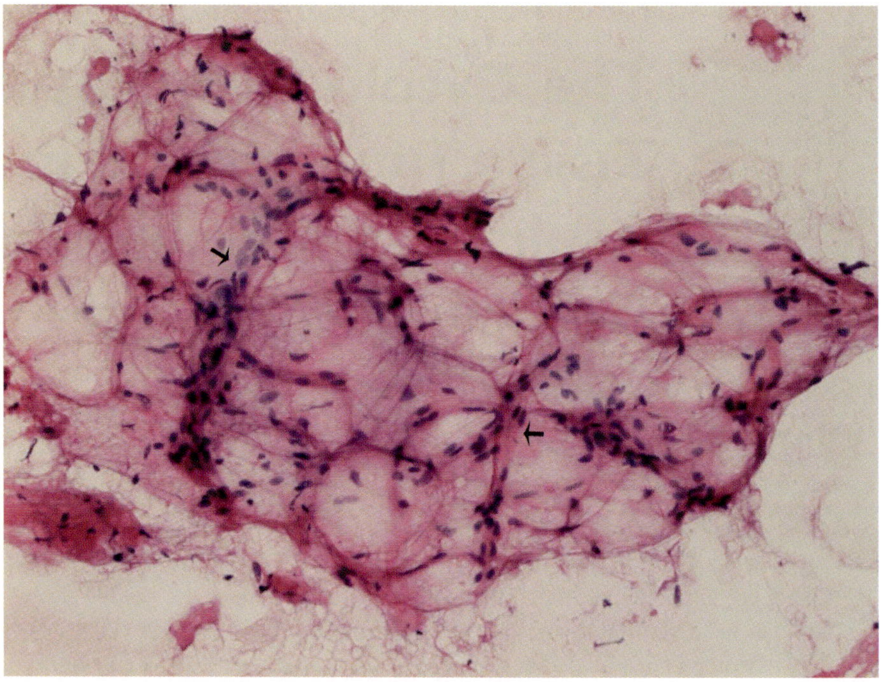

a

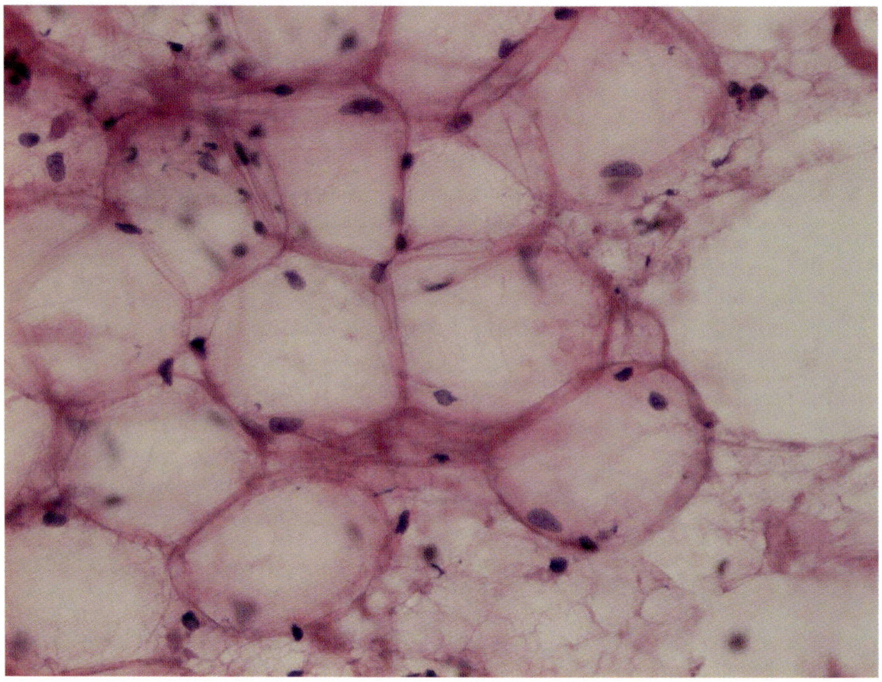

b

Fig. 12. Detail of a smear of a subcutaneous lipoma. **a** Fragment of adipose tissue composed of univacuolated, mature adipocytes. Thin capillaries traverse the fragment (arrows). There are no dissociated adipocytes in the background. HE. Low magnification. **b** Under high power the adipocytes appear as large univacuolated, uniform cells with small, dark nuclei. HE. High magnification.

Myxolipomas have neither the branching capillary network typically seen in smears of myxoid liposarcoma, nor typical lipoblasts.

In lipomas with chondroid metaplasia fragments of chondromyxoid matrix (bluish-bluish-red in MGG) are mixed with the tissue fragments. Chondrocytes may be observed in lacunae in these fragments. Lipomas with chondroid metaplasia have been misdiagnosed as myxoid liposarcoma.

Intramuscular Lipoma

Intramuscular lipoma is a slow-growing tumour. Most are localized in the thigh and trunk. At histological examination intramuscular lipoma is composed of mature fat cells, the adipose tissue infiltrating between muscle fibres. Rarely, intramuscular lipomas may be well circumscribed and not infiltrating.

Cytological features of intramuscular lipoma (fig. 13a, b).

Fragments of large univacuolated, mature adipocytes mixed with more or less atrophic muscle fibres

Multinucleated regenerating muscle fibres ('muscle giant cells') may be observed

Comments

Smears from subcutaneous lipoma may contain inadvertently aspirated normal muscle fibres if the needle is inserted too deeply. The presence of 'muscle giant cells' is the best evidence that the smears are derived from an intramuscular lipoma. Smears from an intramuscular haemangioma can occasionally mimic those from an intramuscular lipoma since atrophic muscle fibres adjacent to haemangioma can be replaced by fat tissue.

Angiolipoma

Angiolipomas are almost always subcutaneous, often multiple and not seldom painful or tender. The majority are smaller than 2 cm.

Histopathology

Angiolipomas are encapsulated and composed of a mixture of mature fat cells and a branching network of small vessels. The vascular channels characteristically contain fibrin thrombi. Some angiolipomas consist almost entirely of the vascular channels. Mast cells are often numerous in angiolipoma.

Cytological features of angiolipoma (fig. 14)

Aggregates or strands of thighly packed small vessels in the fat tissue fragments

Occasionally fibrin thrombi in individual vessels

Variable number of mast cells

Spindle Cell and Pleomorphic Lipoma

These two examples of benign lipoma variants share clinical, morphological and cytogenetic features. They may be essentially the same tumour, but lying at the extremes of a morphological spectrum.

Both are slowly growing and occur typically in the subcutaneous tissue of middle-aged men, most frequently in the upper back, the neck and over the shoulders.

Rare cases can be seen in the head and neck region, including the mouth. Both variants exhibit the same chromosomal aberration, involving the long arm of chromosomes 13 and 16 (monosomy 16 with or without partial loss of 16q).

Spindle cell lipoma

Histopathology

There is a variable mixture of mature fat and fascicles or rows of bland spindle cells in a variably myxoid stroma. Brightly eosinophilic hyaline collagen fibres are a typical feature. A variable number of mast cells is seen. The spindle cells are strongly positive for CD34.

The cytological features of spindle cell lipoma have been published, based on a re-examination of 12 patients [19].

Cytological features of spindle cell lipoma (fig. 15a, b, 16a, b, c)

A mixture of mature adipose tissue and dispersed or clustered, bland-looking spindle cells, often in a myxoid background

Fragments of brightly eosinophilic (HE) collagen-hyaline fibres

Mast cells (particularly when the background is myxoid)

Differential diagnosis

Neurilemoma

Dermatofibrosarcoma protuberans

Low-grade myxofibrosarcoma

Myxoid liposarcoma

Comment

Tumours showing a mixture of spindle cell and pleomorphic lipoma patterns are not uncommon. They most often resemble spindle cell lipomas containing multinucleated cells with hyperchromatic nuclei. Due to the variable proportions of fatty tissue, spindle cells and myxoid background substance, smears of spindle cell lipoma may, in some cases, be misinterpreted as several other types of benign or malignant spindle cell or myxoid tumours. Smears with an abundant myxoid background may easily be misinterpreted as myxoid liposarcoma or low-grade myxofibrosarcoma. Neither the branching network of thin capillaries typical of myxoid liposarcoma, nor the coarse vessel fragments seen in myxofibrosarcoma are, however, present in spindle cell lipoma. The spindle cells in spindle cell lipoma are CD34-positive and S-100-negative, which helps to exclude neurilemoma. As the spindle cells in dermatofibrosarcoma protuberans also are CD34 positive, IC is of no help in this differential diagnosis.

Pleomorphic Lipoma

Histopathology

Pleomorphic lipoma is composed of mature adipocytes mixed with a variable amount of scattered bizarre giant cells with hyperchromatic nuclei and multinucleated large cells with rounded dark nuclei forming rings ('floret cells').

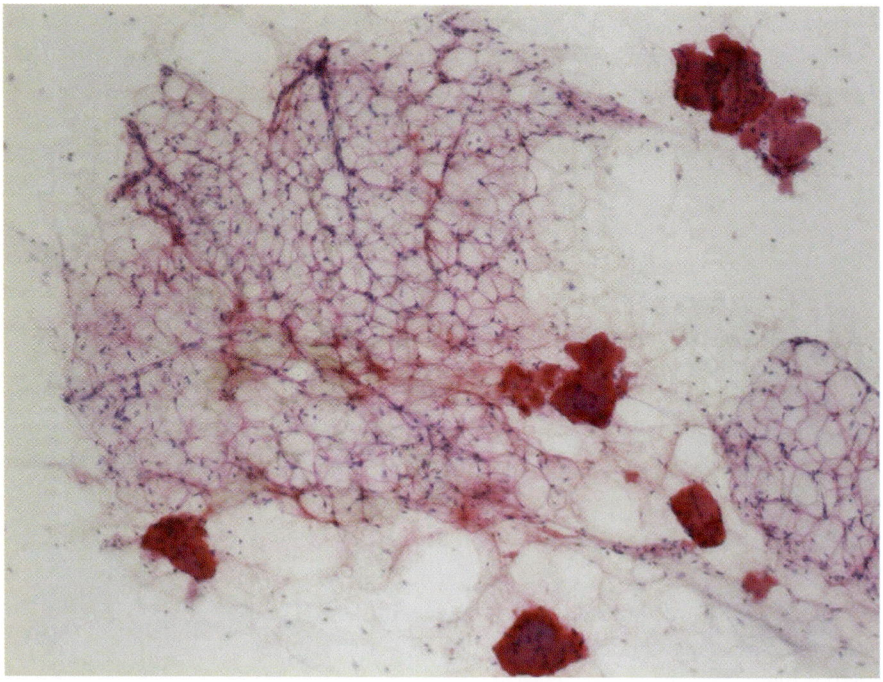

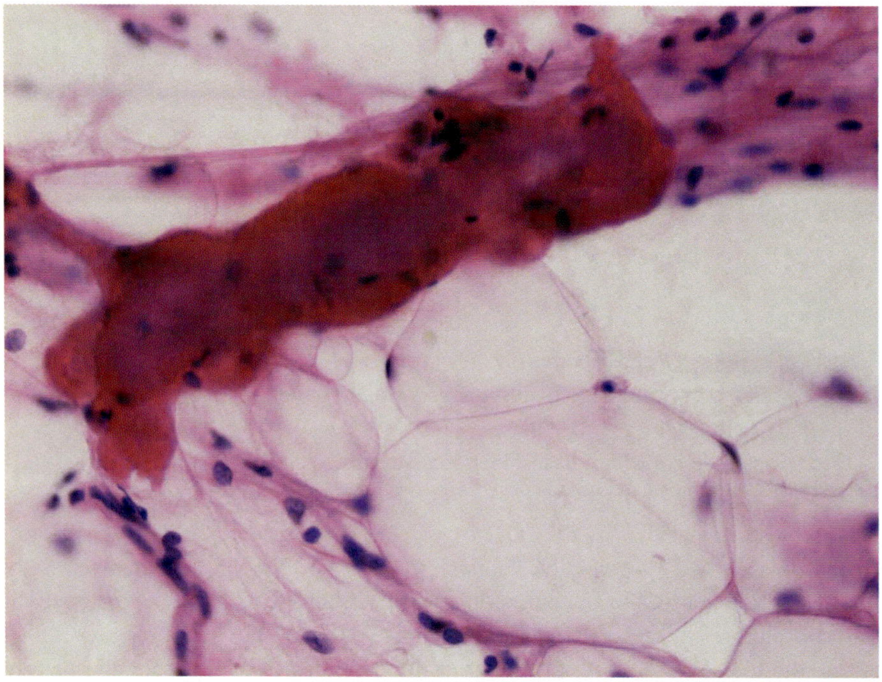

Fig. 13. Intramuscular lipoma. Fragments of adipose tissue composed of mature adipocytes and fragments of striated muscle. **a** Overview, low magnification. **b** High magnification. **a**, **b** HE.

Pleomorphic lipomas may have a myxoid stroma and collagen bundles similar to those in spindle cell lipoma are often present. Transitional forms between pleomorphic and spindle cell lipoma are fairly common. The giant cells stain for CD34.

Cytological features of pleomorphic lipoma (fig. 17a, b)

- Fragments of mature fat
- A variable number of large cells with hyperchromatic nuclei and eosinophilic cytoplasm (HE) both in the background and in tissue fragments
- A variable number of 'floret cells'
- Clusters or runs of spindle cells seen in transitional forms

Differential diagnosis

- Well-differentiated liposarcoma (atypical lipomatous tumour)

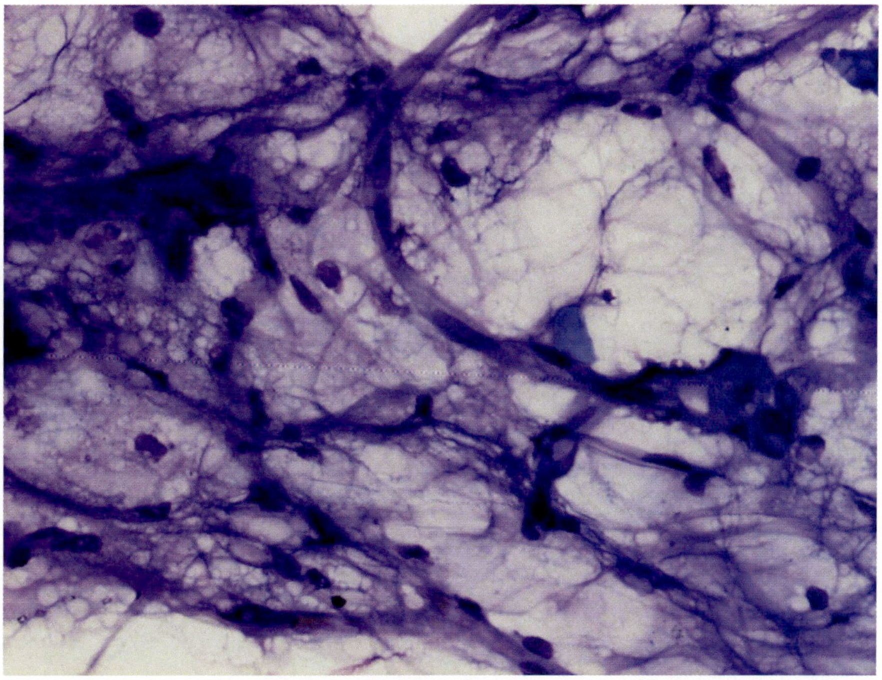

Fig. 14. Smear of angiolipoma. Numerous strands of thin capillary vessels traverse the adipose tissue in every direction. MGG. High magnification.

Comment

The most important differential diagnosis of pleomorphic lipoma is atypical lipomatous tumour/well-differentiated liposarcoma, which often displays large cells with hyperchromatic nuclei and occasional 'floret cells' in smears. The main differences between these two entities are the clinical presentation and the occurrence of atypical lipoblasts in liposarcoma. Pleomorphic lipomas are subcutaneous tumours while atypical lipomatous tumours/well-differentiated liposarcomas usually are deep-seated tumours of the limbs or the retroperitoneum. Cytogenetic findings are also helpful, since atypical lipomatous tumour/well-differentiated liposarcoma typically displays giant marker chromosomes while the pleomorphic lipoma shows involvement of chromosomes 13 and 16, similar to spindle cell lipoma.

Hibernoma

Hibernoma, derived from brown fat, is a rare lipomatous tumour, which occurs mainly in patients between 20 and 50 years of age.

Most hibernomas occur in the back but some in the thigh and in the armpit. Though usually subcutaneous, they can be intramuscular.

Histopathology

Hibernomas are usually well circumscribed and show a tan-brown cut surface. They are lobulated and composed of a variable amount of mature adipocytes mixed with large rounded cells having a finely vacuolated cytoplasm and similar cells with eosinophilic granular cytoplasm. Mature adipocytes are the most common cellular component and may dominate the microscopic picture entirely. Hibernomas are well vascularized. The cytology of hibernoma has been evaluated in case reports and small series [16–18].

Cytological features of hibernoma (fig. 18a, b)

Fragments of mature fat tissue intermingled with 'hibernoma' cells (rounded cells with abundant finely vacuolaed or granular cytoplasm and centrally located, small, uniform nuclei)

The fat fragments often contain numerous capillary vessels

Differential diagnosis

Subcutaneous lipoma

Granular cell tumour

Adult rhabdomyoma

Liposarcoma

Comments

If 'hibernoma cells' dominate the smears, granular cell tumour as well as adult rhabdomyoma can be diagnostic pitfalls. IC is helpful since the cells of granular cell tumour show double positivity for NSA and S-100, and rhabdomyoma cells stain positive for myoglobin. Hibernoma cells have been misinterpreted as lipoblasts but nuclei are neither atypical nor scalloped.

Hibernomas with a large proportion of mature fat cells are often diagnosed as common lipoma.

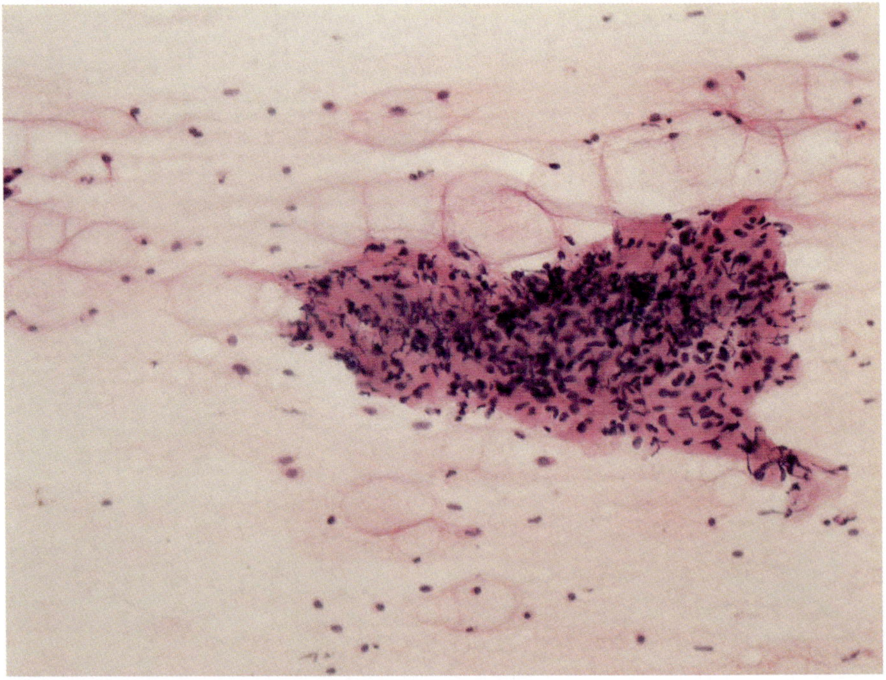

a

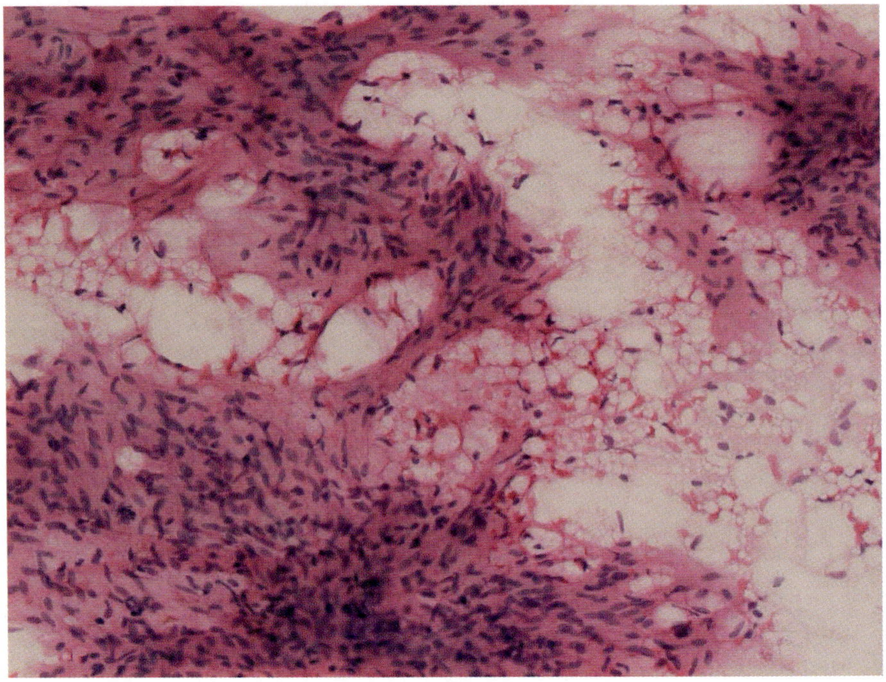

b

Fig. 15. Spindle cell lipoma. The variable proportions of fatty tissue and spindle cells is evident in low magnification. **a**, **b** HE.

Lipoblastoma

Most cases of lipoblastoma are present in infants under the age of 3 years. They have been occasionally reported in children up to 8 years. The majority of lipoblastomas are subcutaneous, well circumscribed and slowly growing. The rare cases of deep-seated, often intramuscular lipoblastomas that are diffusely infiltrative are known as lipoblastomatosis. Individual cases of FNA of lipoblastoma have been published [16, 18].

Histopathology

The lipoblastoma is a lobular tumour composed of a mixture of mature and immature fat cells in varying proportions. A myxoid stroma, lipoblast-like cells, primitive

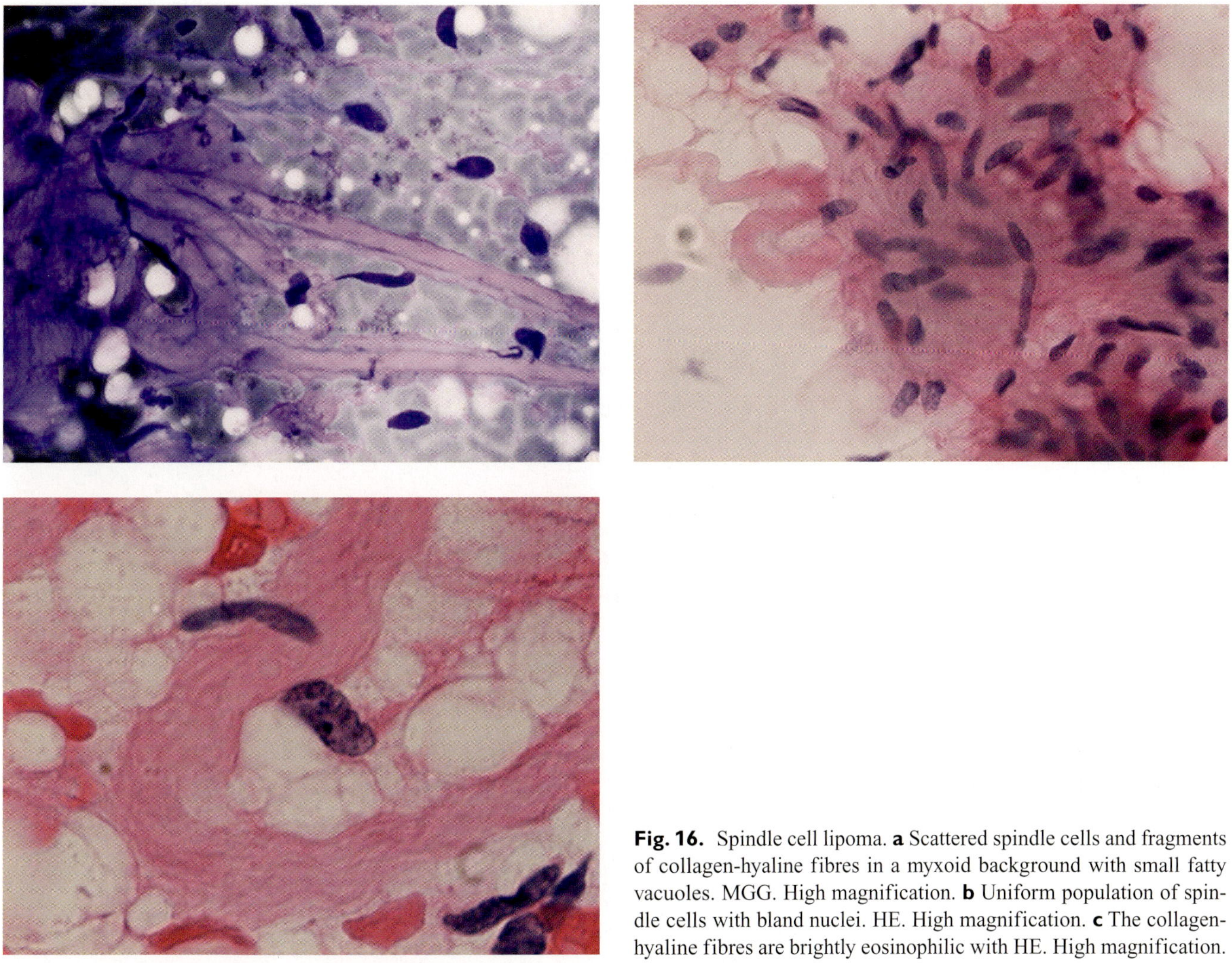

Fig. 16. Spindle cell lipoma. **a** Scattered spindle cells and fragments of collagen-hyaline fibres in a myxoid background with small fatty vacuoles. MGG. High magnification. **b** Uniform population of spindle cells with bland nuclei. HE. High magnification. **c** The collagen-hyaline fibres are brightly eosinophilic with HE. High magnification.

spindle-shaped mesenchymal cells and capillaries are typical features of immature areas of lipoblastoma. The more mature component resembles a common lipoma with occasional hibernoma-like cells. Lipoblastoma may mature towards common lipoma and the characteristic immature areas may be very small and focal.

Cytological features of lipoblastoma (fig. 19a, b)

- Fatty tissue fragments with variable amounts of myxoid background matrix
- Branching strands of thin capillaries
- Uni- or multivacuolated lipoblast-like cells mixed with small and large univacuolated fat cells with uniform nuclei

Differential diagnosis

- Common lipoma
- Myxoid liposarcoma

Comments

The most important pitfall from the cytological point of view is myxoid liposarcoma (myxoid background substance, capillary network, lipoblast-like cells). Myxoid liposarcoma has been described in children under 10 years of age, albeit very rare. The most common error made is to misdiagnose a lipoblastoma as a common lipoma when smears are dominated by ordinary large univacuolated fat cells. The chromosomal aberration, 8q 11–13 seen in lipoblastoma is a reliable diagnostic aid.

Chondroid Lipoma

Chondroid lipoma is a recently described rare variant of benign lipoma. Chondroid lipoma is mainly found in adults between 30 and 40 years of age and is predominantly a subcutaneous lesion in the limbs, trunk, head and neck region.

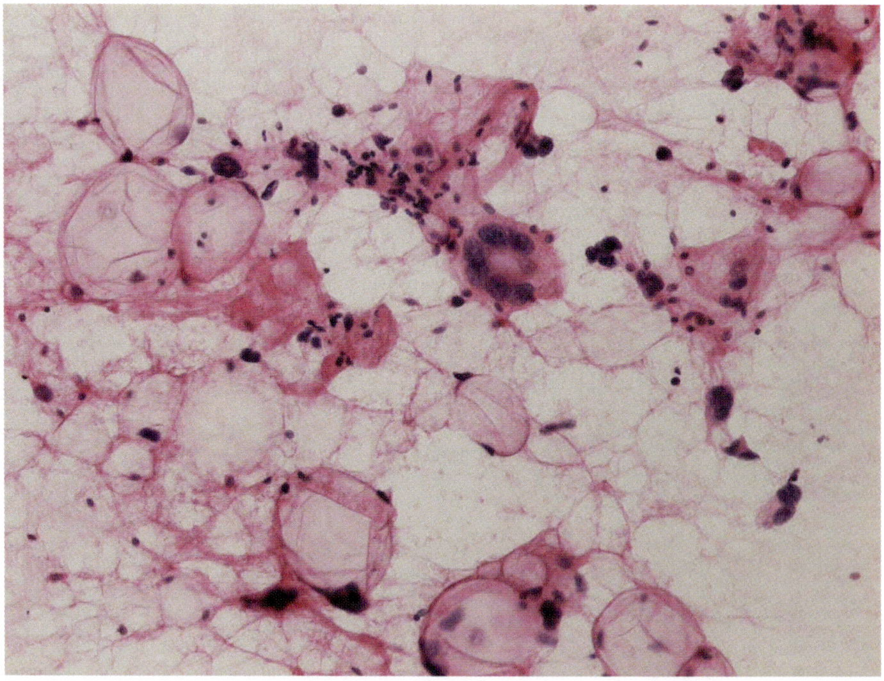

a

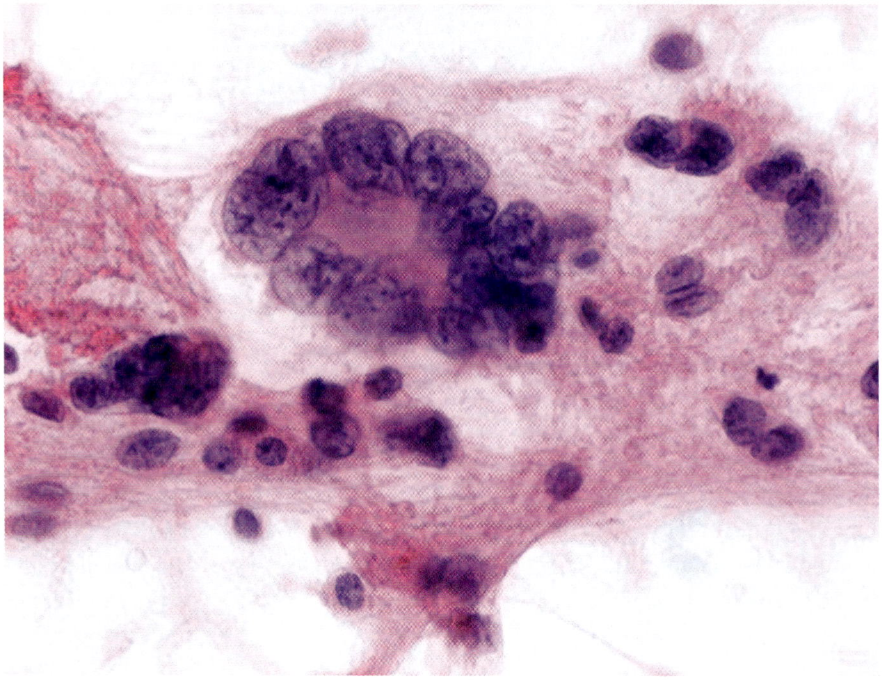

b

Fig. 17. Pleomorphic lipoma. **a** Mature adipocytes, scattered cells with large hyperchromatic nuclei and a single floret cell. HE. Low magnification. **b** Typical floret cell. HE. High magnification.

Histopathology

Chondroid lipoma is a well-demarcated, at times encapsulated tumour. It has a lobular pattern and is composed of rounded cells arranged in nests or strands in a chondroid-like matrix. The tumour cells may resemble multivacuolated lipoblasts, others have an eosinophilic granular cytoplasm. Foci of mature fat cells are also present. The nuclei are often irregular with a folded nuclear membrane.

The cytological features of chondroid lipoma are described in FNA smears based on individual cases [70, 71].

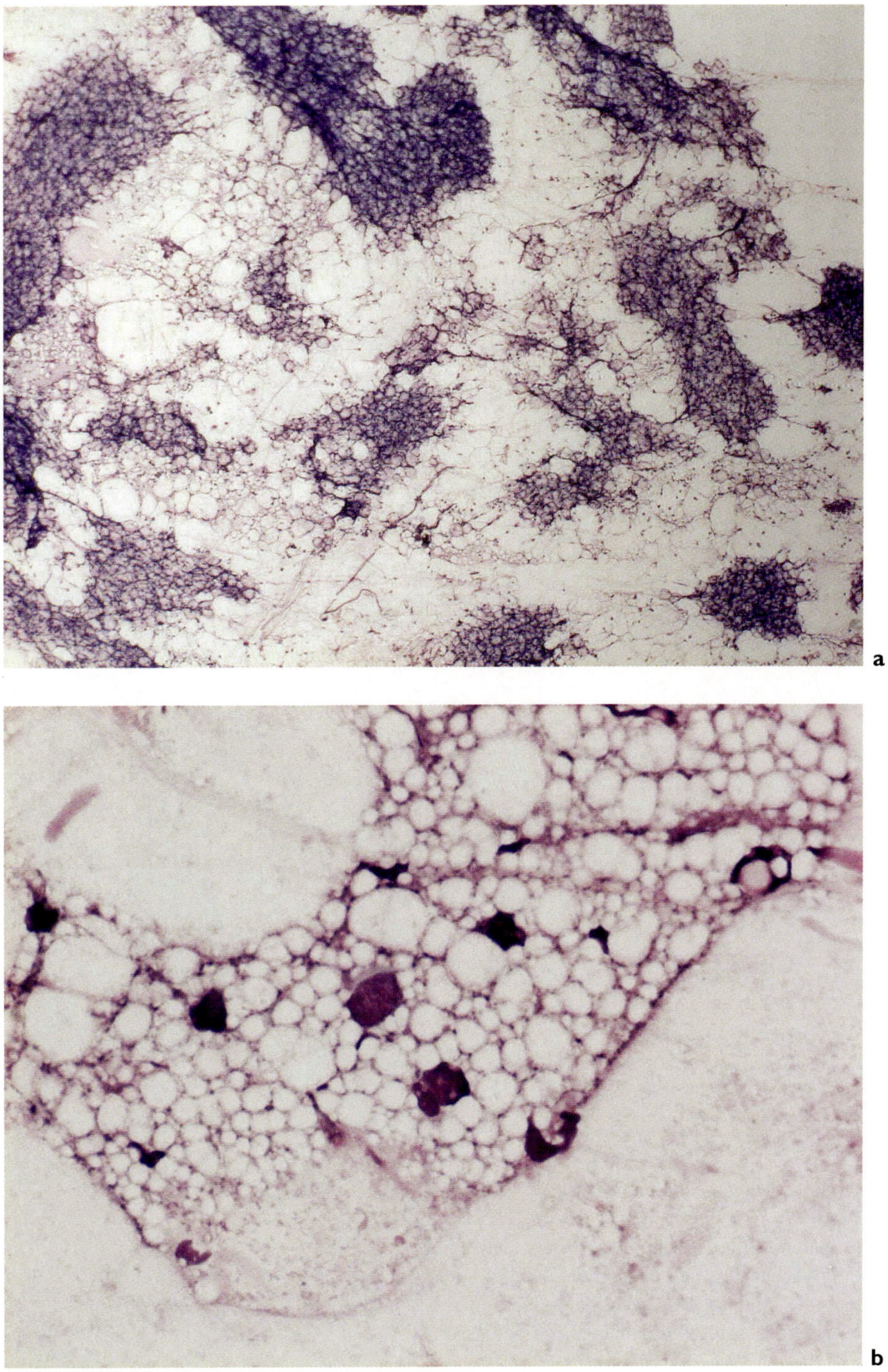

Fig. 18. Hibernoma. **a** The typical mixture of mature fat and clusters of 'hibernoma' cells is evident under low power. MGG. Low magnification. **b** The 'hibernoma' cells have an abundant finely vacuolated cytoplasm and centrally located uniform nuclei. MGG. High magnification.

Cytological features of chondroid lipoma (fig. 20a–d)

- Variable amount of myxo-chondroid background matrix
- Clusters or groups of mature large adipocytes mixed with clusters or groups of uni- or multivacuolated lipoblast-like cells
- Lipoblast-like cells have irregular nuclei of varying sizes, often lobulated or grooved
- Chondrocyte-like cells sometimes seen in the background matrix

Differential diagnosis

- Myxoid liposarcoma
- Extraskeletal myxoid chondrosarcoma

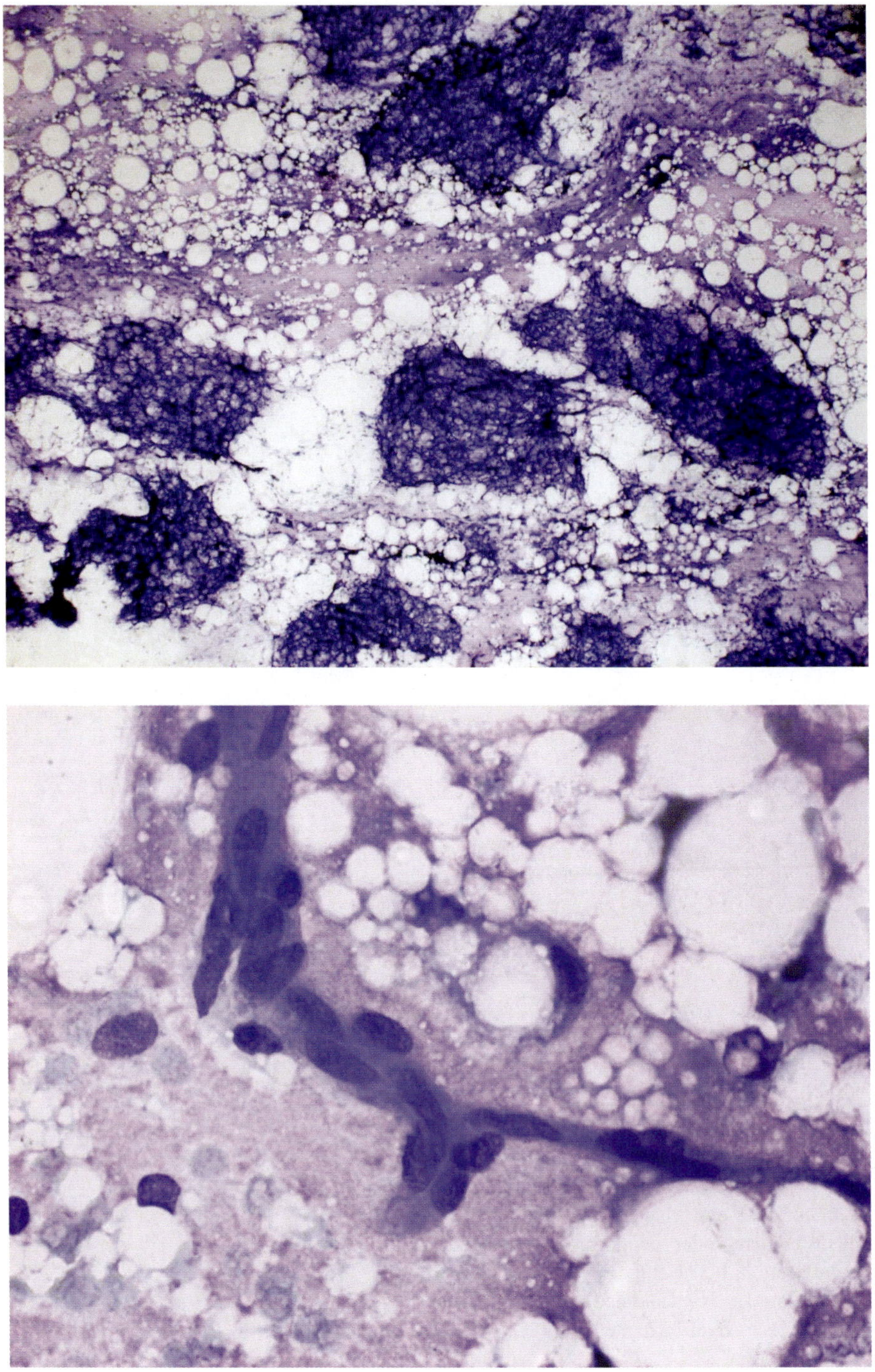

a

b

Fig. 19. Lipoblastoma. **a** Myxoid background with fatty vacuoles and fragments of tightly packed small fat cells. MGG. Low magnification. **b** A thin capillary strand in a myxoid background surrounded by lipoblast-like cells. MGG. High magnification.

Comments

In the few cases hitherto described, the branching capillary network seen in myxoid liposarcoma has not been present. In addition the myxoid matrix is less abundant and the nuclei of the lipoblast-like cells are more irregular compared to the rounded, slightly atypical nuclei seen in myxoid liposarcoma.

Extra-Adrenal Myelolipoma

Extra-adrenal myelolipoma, a tumour-like lesion composed of mature fat and bone marrow cells, is mainly found in the adrenals. These lesions may also arise in the pelvic region and retroperitoneum. In cytological practice myelolipoma is part of the differential diagnostic spectrum when tumour-like masses in the pelvic region or retroperitoneum are needled [72].

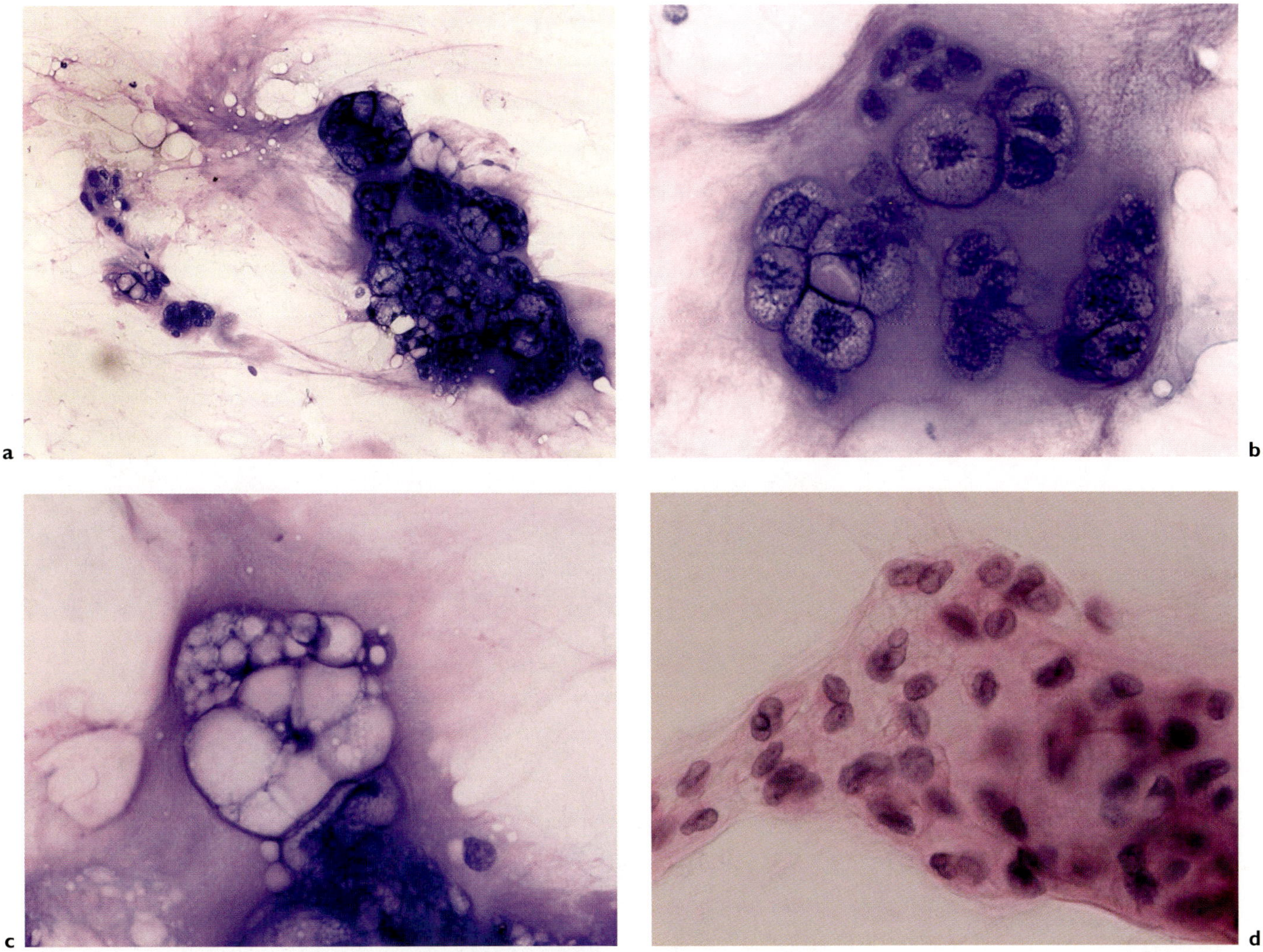

Fig. 20. Chondroid lipoma. **a** Low power view of groups of vacuolated cells with a partly myxoid, partly fatty background. MGG. Low magnification. **b** A group of chondroblast-like cells in a myxohyaline background. MGG. High magnification. **c** Lipoblast-like cells. MGG. High magnification. **d** Wet-fixed smear showing irregular nuclei with folded nuclear membranes. HE. High magnification.

The histogenesis of myelolipoma is not clarified. One hypothesis is that myelolipoma originates from rests of haematopoietic stem cells.

Histopathology

Myelolipomas are composed of a mixture of mature fat cells and bone marrow cells in varying proportions. The bone marrow elements consist of erythropoietic and myelopoietic cells and megakaryocytes.

Cytological features of myelolipoma (fig. 21a, b)

- Mature fat cells and normal bone marrow cells in varying proportions
- Often possible to identify bone marrow cells from all three haematopoietic lines

Comment

FNA smears from a myelolipoma do not differ microscopically from smears obtained from bone marrow of the pelvic bones. It is thus important to make sure that the needle has sampled a soft tissue mass and not bone. Most often a myelolipoma is an incidental finding on a CT scan or MRI in the investigation of abdominal pain or discomfort.

Liposarcoma

Liposarcoma is one of the most common soft tissue sarcomas. It has been estimated that about 20% of soft tissue sarcomas in adults are liposarcoma. In the Central Soft

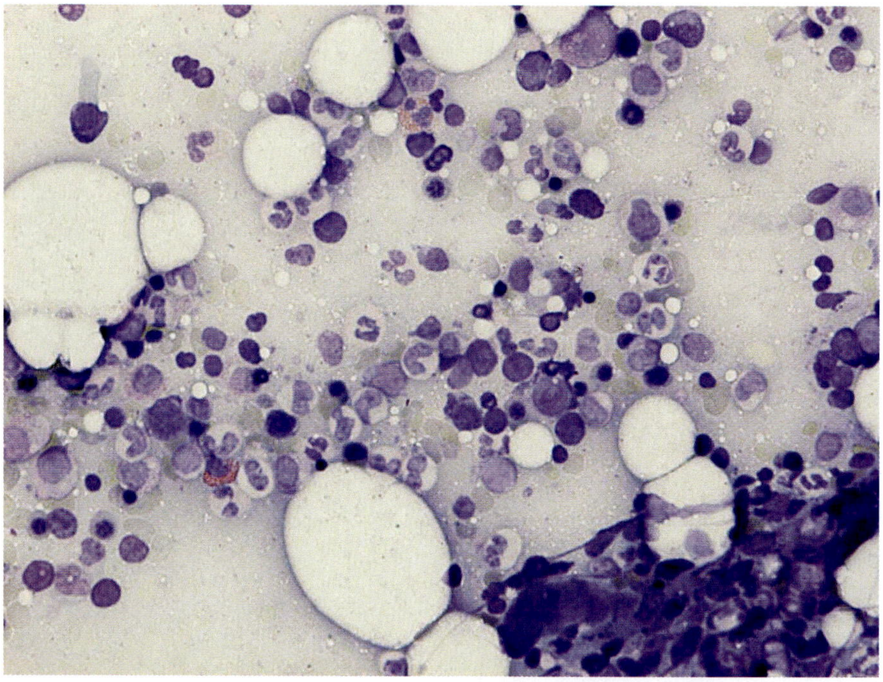

a

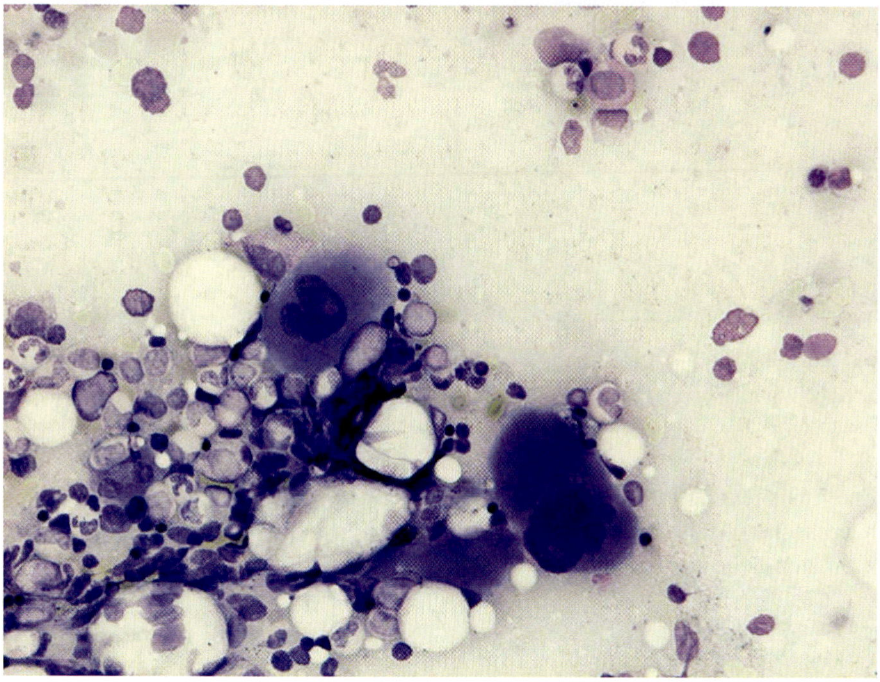

b

Fig. 21. Extra-adrenal myelolipoma. **a**, **b** Mature fat cells and numerous haematopoietic cells. All three lineages are evident. MGG. Low magnification.

Tissue Sarcoma Registry of the Scandinavian Sarcoma Group (a multidisciplinary group with members from all Nordic countries) liposarcoma was the third most common sarcoma.

The majority of liposarcomas are deep-seated, intra- or intermuscular, and the most common sites are the extremities, trunk and retroperitoneum.

Three large groups of liposarcomas are identified: well-differentiated/dedifferentiated, myxoid/round cell, and pleomorphic.

Well-Differentiated and Dedifferentiated Liposarcoma

Well-differentiated liposarcoma occurs most commonly in late adult life (age 60–70). About 75% are intramuscular tumours of the extremities, up to 25% develop in the retroperitoneum and of the remaining cases the groin and spermatic cord are the most frequent sites. Subcutaneous tumours may occur in the extremities but are rare. Three subtypes of well-differentiated liposarcoma have been recognized: lipoma-like, sclerosing and inflammatory. Mixed forms are often diagnosed. Well-differentiated liposarcoma is considered to be a non-metastasizing tumour and is diagnosed as a low-grade sarcoma. Limb tumours have a low recurrence rate while retroperitoneal tumours often recur and may dedifferentiate to a high-grade sarcoma with metastasizing capabilities. It is estimated that 10–15% of retroperitoneal tumours dedifferentiate while limb tumours, mainly intramuscular tumours, dedifferentiate in 5–6%. Based on this site-dependent behaviour it has been suggested that the term atypical lipoma should be used for the limb tumours but the retroperitoneal tumours should be diagnosed as liposarcoma.

The World Health Organization has suggested that the rare subcutaneous tumours should be diagnosed as atypical lipoma, the deep-seated limb tumours as well-differentiated liposarcoma/atypical lipoma and the retroperitoneal tumours as well-differentiated liposarcoma [73]. Kempson et al. [1] have proposed a different terminology: atypical lipomatous tumour including atypical lipoma and well-differentiated liposarcoma. The histological features are the same irrespective of site as is the typical cytogenetic aberration (giant marker and ring chromosomes).

Histopathology

There is a predominance of mature fat cells combined with a variable amount of atypical cells with irregular hyperchromatic nuclei and multivacuolated lipoblasts. The lipoblasts are usually infrequent. The atypical cells are either situated among the mature fat cells or in fibrotic strands or trabeculae, and are also commonly seen in the perivascular tissue or within the vessel walls.

Cytological features of well-differentiated liposarcoma (fig. 22a–d)

A predominance of mature fat cells arranged in clusters or sheets

Variable presence of fusiform, rounded or polygonal, large atypical cells with irregular hyperchromatic nuclei

Rare multivacuolated lipoblasts

Variable presence of fragments of fibrous tissue with atypical cells

Differential diagnosis

Lipoma

Fat necrosis with lipophages

Comment

We suggest that the term atypical lipomatous tumour proposed by Kempson et al. [1] for these tumours be used by cytologists. As many atypical lipomatous tumours may include large areas of lipoma-like tissue, extensive sampling from large tumours, especially intra-abdominal tumours, is important.

The cytoplasm of lipophages in fat necrosis is usually foamy or filled with small vacuoles. The nuclei are rather small and not indented (scalloped).

Dedifferentiated Liposarcoma

Histopathology

The dedifferentiated areas in well-differentiated liposarcoma are often sharply demarcated and predominantly composed of atypical spindle cells resembling a fibrosarcoma or of a pleomorphic cellular population like that found in pleomorphic sarcoma of the malignant fibrous histiocytoma (MFH) type.

Cytological features of dedifferentiated liposarcoma

Highly atypical spindly or pleomorphic sarcoma cells, dispersed or in clusters or groups

Variable numbers of clusters or groups of mature fat cells

Differential diagnosis

High-grade spindle or pleomorphic sarcoma of another lineage

Comment

The cytological diagnosis of dedifferentiated liposarcoma is based on the presence of mature fat cells and a highly atypical cellular population. As these tumours are often large it is important to collect material from various areas, especially from sites which are considered non-lipomatous by radiographic imaging.

Myxoid/Round Cell Liposarcoma

About 50% of liposarcomas are diagnosed as myxoid/round cell liposarcoma. These two variants share the same cytogenetic abnormality: t(12;16)(q13;p11) with fusion of the CHOP gene on chromosome 12 with the TLS gene on chromosome 16.

Myxoid Liposarcoma

Histopathology

Myxoid liposarcomas are multilobulated tumours with an abundant myxoid matrix. A plexiform capillary vessel network is a typical finding and cellularity is rather low. The tumour cell population is composed of both spindle cells and

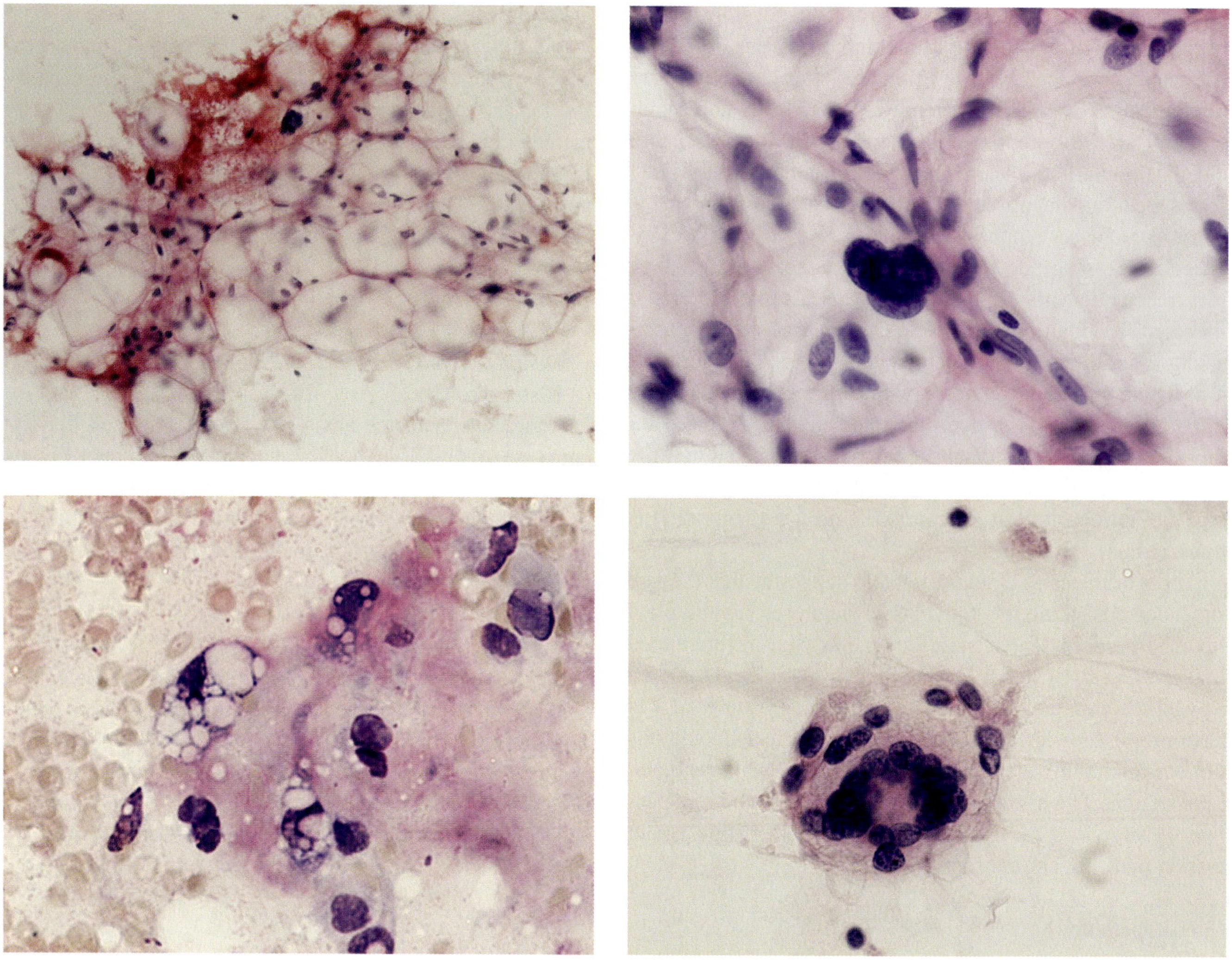

Fig. 22. Well-differentiated liposarcoma (atypical lipomatous tumour). **a** Scattered large cells with hyperchromatic nuclei within a fragment of mature adipose tissue. HE. Low magnification. **b** The atypical cells often have irregular, hyperchromatic nuclei. HE. High magnification. **c** Multivacuolated lipoblasts may be present but are not necessary for the diagnosis. MGG. High magnification. **d** Multinucleated floret cells may also be present in well-differentiated liposarcoma. HE. High magnification.

uni- or multivacuolated lipoblasts. Cellular atypia is moderate and mitoses are few. Myxoid liposarcoma has been fairly extensively described in FNA material [16, 17, 32].

Cytological features of myxoid liposarcoma (fig. 23a–c)

Abundant myxoid matrix
Variable number of vacuolated tumour tissue fragments with a branching network of capillary vessels
Few or no dispersed tumour cells
Uni- or multivacuolated lipoblasts within tissue fragments, especially alongside capillary vessels
Spindly or rounded tumour cells other than lipoblasts
Slight to moderate nuclear atypia
No mitotic figures

Differential diagnosis

Spindle cell lipoma with abundant myxoid matrix
Intramuscular myxoma
Low-grade myxofibrosarcoma

Comment

The clue to the diagnosis of myxoid liposarcoma is the diagnostic triad of a background of abundant myxoid matrix, fragments of tumour tissue with a branching network of thin capillaries, and slightly atypical lipoblasts in fragments often along the capillary vessels.

The presence of vessels in the smears and their site and size are important diagnostic criteria. In intramuscular myxoma only scattered vessel fragments are present in the

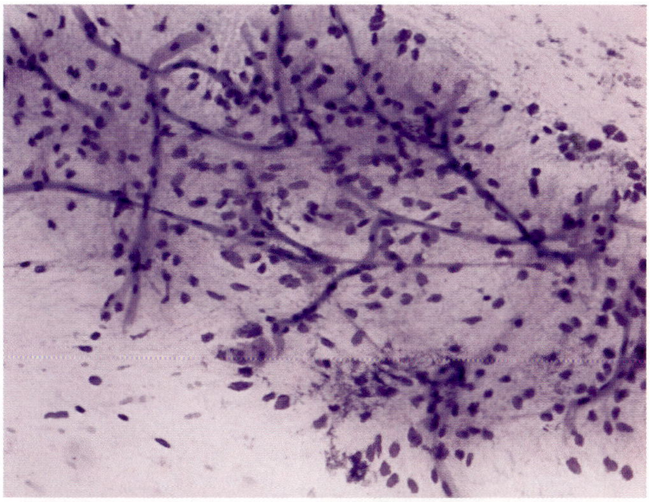

a

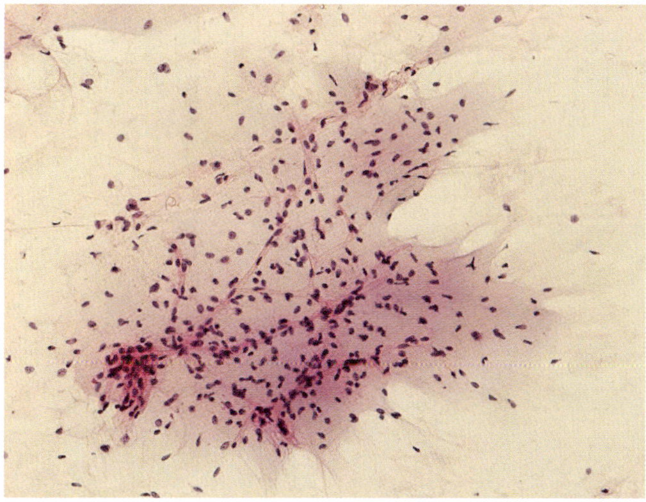

b

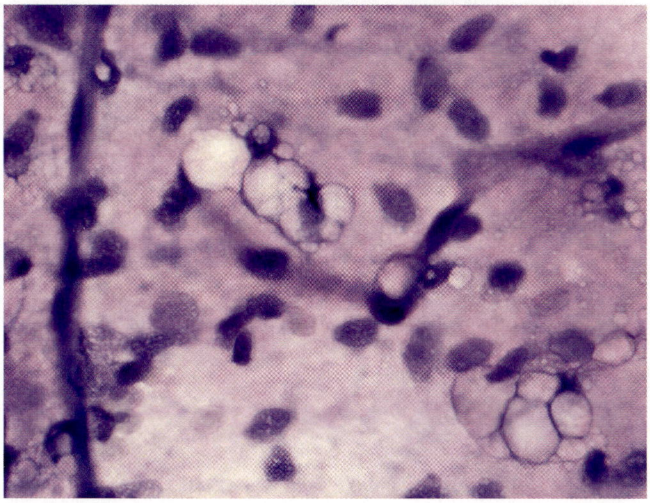

c

Fig. 23. Myxoid liposarcoma. **a** Low power view showing the typical appearance of myxoid liposarcoma. MGG. Low magnification. **b** Another low power view stained with HE. Note that the myxoid background is less evident. Low magnification. **c** This high power view shows a capillary network, multivacuolated lipoblasts and rounded tumour cells embedded in myxoid matrix. MGG. High magnification.

myxoid background. The vessel fragments in myxofibrosarcoma are found in the background matrix and are nonbranching coarse fragments.

Round cell Liposarcoma

Histopathology

Pure round cell liposarcoma or foci of round cell liposarcoma in myxoid liposarcoma are composed of sheets of rounded cells with scanty cytoplasm and rounded, atypical nuclei often with nucleoli. The myxoid background is less evident or absent. Atypical lipoblasts are present among the tumour cells but may be difficult to identify.

Cytological features of round cell liposarcoma (fig. 24a, b)

Variable proportions of dispersed tumour cells and highly cellular tumour fragments
Stripped nuclei common
Myxoid matrix and capillary network less conspicuous than in myxoid liposarcoma
Rounded tumour cells with scanty cytoplasm and rounded nuclei with irregular chromatin
Atypical lipoblasts
Mitoses may be found

Differential diagnosis

Other types of round cell sarcoma infiltrating adipose tissue
Soft tissue metastasis of renal carcinoma

Comment

True round cell liposarcomas are rare. Most are composed of both typical myxoid liposarcoma tissue and highly cellular areas as described above. In histopathology the terms paucicellular and cellular myxoid liposarcoma, respectively, have been proposed instead of myxoid and round cells. The metastatic potential is increased if 25% or

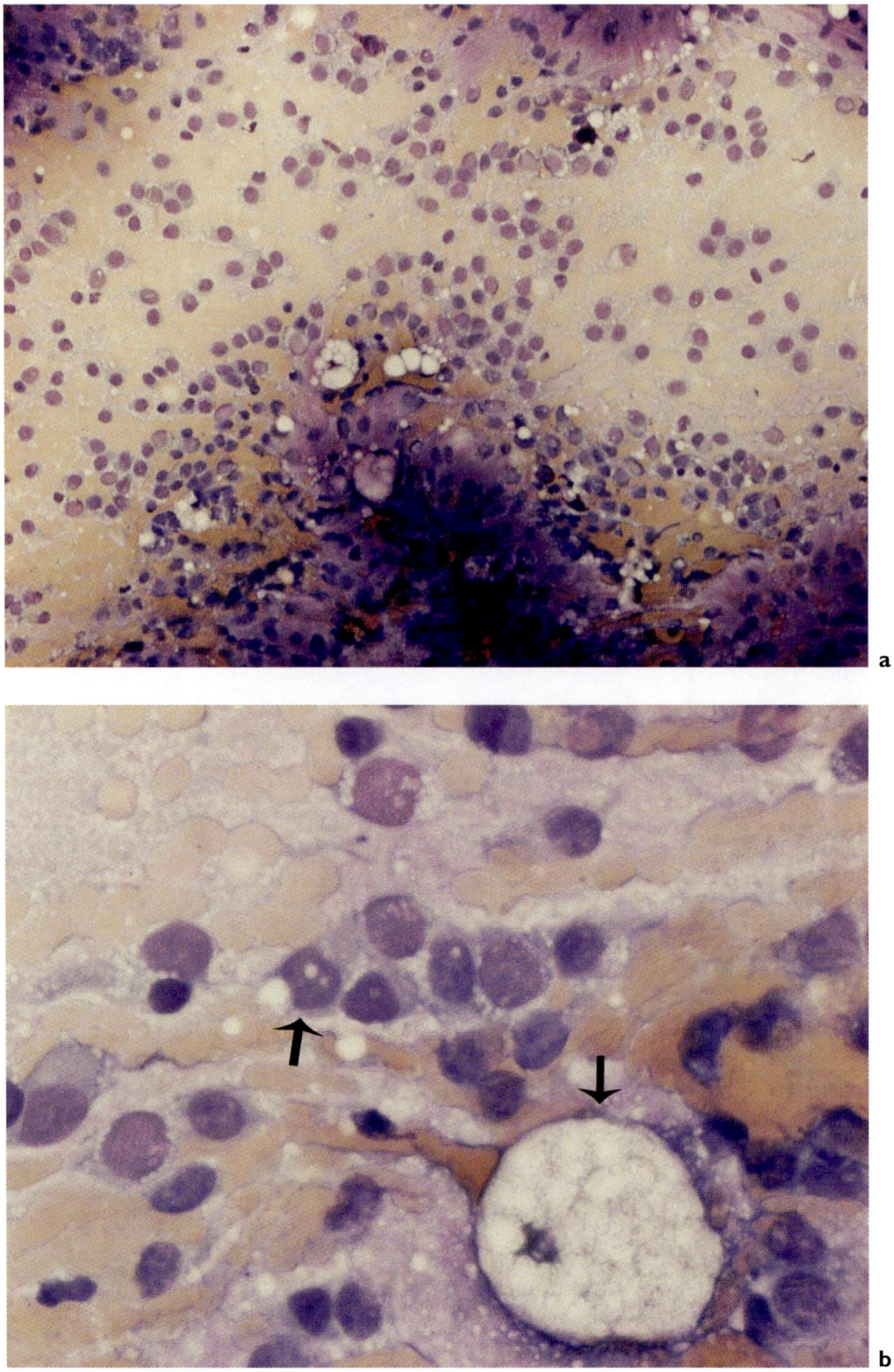

Fig. 24. Pure round cell liposarcoma. **a** Predominantly dissociated tumour cells with rounded nuclei in a myxoid background. MGG. Low magnification. **b** Scattered lipoblasts seen in high magnification (arrows). MGG.

more of the tumour is cellular [1]. If several parts of the tumour are sampled with FNA, most often a paucicellular and cellular mixture is found.

If unequivocal atypical lipoblasts are difficult to identify, a specific diagnosis of round cell liposarcoma should be avoided.

Pleomorphic Liposarcoma

Histopathology

Pleomorphic liposarcoma is a high-grade sarcoma exhibiting marked atypia. Highly atypical lipoblasts, often multinucleated, are more or less numerous. Hyaline cytoplasmic droplets may be seen in the large atypical cells.

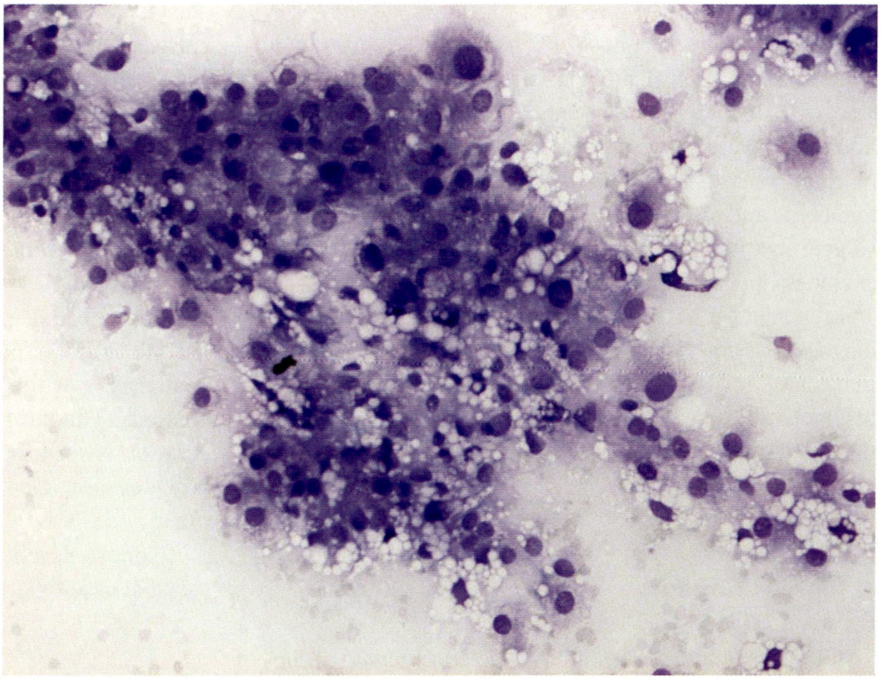

a

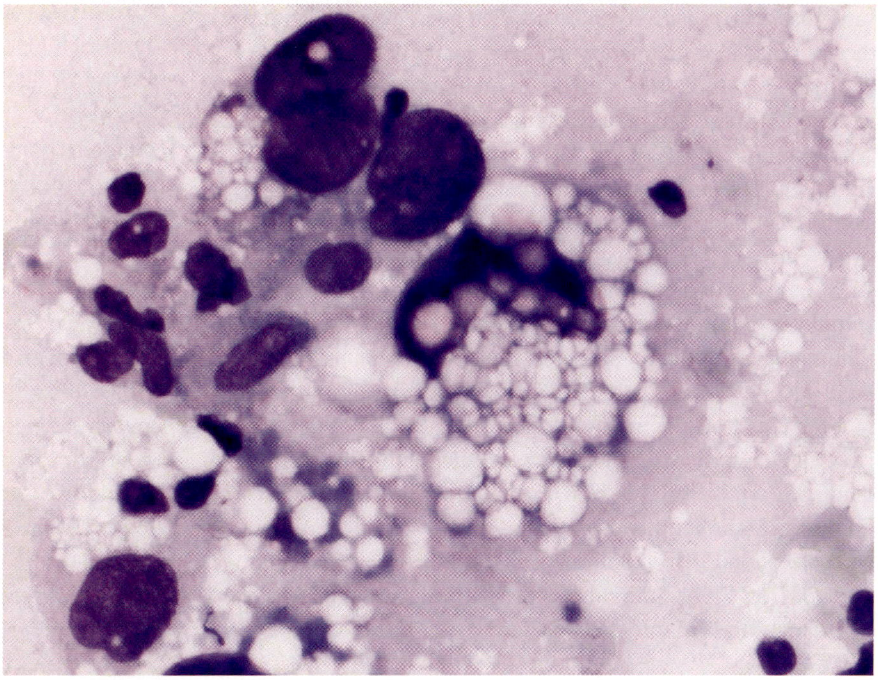

b

Fig. 25. Pleomorphic liposarcoma. **a** Detail of smear of a pleomorphic liposarcoma with unusually large numbers of atypical lipoblasts. MGG. Low magnification. **b** High power view of highly atypical lipoblasts in a pleomorphic liposarcoma. MGG.

Cytological features of pleomorphic liposarcoma (fig. 25a, b)

Dispersed cells and cell clusters

Necrosis commonly seen in fragments

Pleomorphic tumour cells, including multinucleated giant tumour cells

Variable presence of highly atypical uni- or multinucleated lipoblasts

Variable presence of tumour cells with multiple hyaline cytoplasmic droplets

Differential diagnosis

Pleomorphic high-grade sarcoma of another lineage

Comment

For a specific diagnosis of pleomorphic liposarcoma, unequivocal atypical lipoblasts must be present in the smears. If lipoblasts are absent, smears from a pleomorphic liposarcoma are impossible to distinguish from other pleomorphic sarcomas such as the malignant fibrous histiocytoma type and pleomorphic leiomyosarcoma. IC is of limited value; positive staining for desmin, SMA or caldesmon excludes liposarcoma.

In general EM is of limited value in the differential diagnosis of adipocytic tumours. Cytogenetic and/or molecular genetic investigations are valuable adjuncts in histopathology. A summary of the cytomorphology of lipomatous tumours and their cytogenetic aberrations is listed in tables 5 and 6.

Fibrous Tumours

Fibrous tumours constitute a heterogeneous group of reactive and hamartomatous lesions, benign tumours and sarcomas. The most frequently needled benign conditions are the 'pseudosarcomatous lesions', especially nodular fasciitis and desmoid tumours, of the sarcomas myxofibrosarcoma and pleomorphic sarcoma of malignant fibrous histiocytoma type are the most common. Elastofibroma and solitary fibrous tumour are, in our experience, occasionally needled as fibrosarcoma and low-grade fibromyxoid sarcoma. The experience of FNA is incomplete in relation to rare sarcomas such as sclerosing epithelioid fibrosarcoma, hyalinizing spindle cell tumour with giant rosettes and acral myxoinflammatory fibroblastic sarcoma. It is non-existent or incomplete also in several of the relatively rare benign fibrous tumours such as fibroma of tendon sheath, collagenous fibroma, angiomyofibroblastoma, cellular angiofibroma and giant cell angiofibroma, based at most on individual cases. Of the vast number of fibrous lesions and tumours in infancy and childhood, fibromatosis colli is the most common referred for FNA. Individual cases of fibrous hamartoma of infancy and infantile fibrosarcoma are also recorded in our files.

Benign Tumours

Nodular Fasciitis

Nodular fasciitis is most often seen in young adults and children. Most are subcutaneous, and common sites are the arms, trunk, head and neck. Nodular fasciitis is a rapidly growing lesion, usually painful and tender. Due to the clinical history most nodular fasciitis lesions are needled in an early phase. The vast majority regress spontaneously and conservative follow-up is the appropriate management if the combined evaluation of clinical data and cytological features is typical [74, 75].

Histopathology

The cells of nodular fasciitis are (myo)fibroblasts showing more or less marked anisocytosis and anisokaryosis. Multinucleated ganglion cell-like myofibroblasts are part of the cellular spectrum. The cells are arranged in various patterns: storiform, whorled or vascularized tissue culture pattern. The stroma is variably myxoid and cystic degeneration is seen. Inflammatory cells and extravasated erythrocytes are a common finding. Mitoses are commonly seen.

Nodular fasciitis in FNA smears have been described in several case reports and a single series [13].

Cytological features of nodular fasciitis (fig. 26a–d)
- More or less abundant myxoid background matrix
- Often rich cellular yield
- Mixture of dispersed cells and cell clusters
- Pleomorphic population of (myo)fibroblasts; spindly, rounded, triangular or polygonal
- Often cytoplasmic processes
- Ganglion cell-like uni- or binucleated cells with eccentric nuclei
- Multinucleated giant cells
- Occasional (frequent) mitoses
- Bland nuclear chromatin but often prominent nucleoli
- Admixture of inflammatory cells

Differential diagnosis
- Myxofibrosarcoma
- Myxoid leiomyosarcoma

Comment

The typical cellular smear showing nuclear pleomorphism, prominent nucleoli and occasional mitoses may suggest a myxoid sarcoma but the bland nuclear chromatin favours a benign process.

The related pseudosarcomatous lesions, proliferative fasciitis and proliferative myositis, share many cytological features with nodular fasciitis. However, the myxoid background matrix is less prominent and the ganglion cell-like cells are numerous and often exhibit large nucleoli (fig. 27). In proliferative myositis the fibroblastic/myofibroblastic proliferation often includes multinucleated regenerating muscle fibres.

Table 5. Cytological features in benign lipomatous tumours and liposarcoma

	Cytological features	Notes
Benign lipomatous tumour		
Common lipoma	Clusters and fragments of adipose tissue with large, univacuolated, mature fat cells with small, dark, eccentric nuclei; variable presence of vessels in fragments; few or no fat cells between fragments	
Intramuscular lipoma	As common lipoma and fragments of striated muscle fibres; occasionally 'muscle giant cells'	
Angiolipoma	Variably cellular fat tissue fragments or clusters, cellularity due to the presence of clustered capillaries; occasionally fibrin thrombin vessels; variable number of mast cells	
Pleomorphic lipoma	Within and outside fat tissue fragments with mature fat cells variable presence of different-sized atypical cells with dark, irregular, at times multinucleated nuclei (floret cells)	Diagnostic site: subcutaneous in neck, shoulder region and back; in other sites tumours with the same cytomorphology should be classified as atypical lipomatous tumours
Spindle cell lipoma	Variable proportions of clustered or dispersed univacuolated, mature fat cells, spindle cells with bland nuclei, and fragments of collagen fibres in a variably myxoid background; the clusters or dissociated mature fat cells may be in minority	Typical site: subcutaneous in neck, shoulder region and back; tumours with features of pleomorphic and spindle cell lipoma not uncommon
Hibernoma	Clusters and fragments of large univacuolate, mature fat cells mixed with variable proportions of 'hibernoma cells' (multivacuolated or granulated cytoplasm); capillary network in clusters and fragments; occasionally dissociated or small groups of hibernoma cells between clusters; aspirates may be dominated by large mature fat cells	
Lipoblastoma	Fat tissue fragments/clusters with variable areas of myxoid background; network of thin capillaries in fragments/clusters; in fragments/clusters variable proportions of mature fat cells and lipoblast-like cells	Usually in infants and children under the age of 3 years
Chondroid lipoma	Clusters of mature fat cells, variable amount of myxochondroid background matrix with rows, groups of lipoblast-like cells with irregular nuclear contours	
Extra-adrenal myelolipoma	Mature fat cells and bone marrow cells in varying proportions	
Liposarcoma		
Well-differentiated liposarcoma/atypical lipomatous tumour	Fragments/clusters of mature fat cells and variable presence of large atypical cells with irregular dark nuclei within and outside fragments/clusters; occasionally lipoblast-like cells	
Dedifferentiated liposarcoma	The same features as above and a cellular population corresponding to high-grade malignant sarcoma, spindle cell, pleomorphic or mixed	Diagnosis of dedifferentiated liposarcoma is based on the presence of material from well-differentiated liposarcoma and high-grade sarcoma in the same smear

Table 5 (continued)

	Cytological features	Notes
Myxoid liposarcoma	Fragments of fat tissue with a distinct network of thin capillaries, slightly atypical spindle cells and uni- or multivacuolated slightly atypical lipoblasts; myxoid back-ground matrix; few dissociated tumour cells	
Round cell liposarcoma	Mixture of dispersed or clustered rounded, atypical cells with rounded nuclei; variable amount of atypical lipoblasts; variabe amount of myxoid background and capillary fragments in clusters; stripped nuclei; mitoses	Pure round cell liposarcoma rare; mixed forms (myxoid and round cell common)
Pleomorphic liposarcoma	Pleomorphic tumour cell population; dispersed cells and small clusters/groups of tumour cells; variable presence of highly atypical, often multinucleated lipoblasts; necrosis	

Table 6. Chromosomal aberrations in lipomatous tumours

Lipomatous tumour	Chromosomal aberrations	Genes involved
Common lipoma	Translocations involving 12q13–15 Rearrangements involving 6p21–33 Rearrangements of 13q	
Pleomorphic/spindle cell lipoma	Monosomy 16 or partial loss of 16q associated with unbalanced aberration at 13q	
Lipoblastoma	Rearrangements involving 8q11–13	
Hibernoma	Rearrangements involving 11q13;10q22	
Well-differentiated liposarcoma/atypical lipomatous tumour	Ring chromosomes, long marker chromosomes from 12q13–15	
Myxoid/round cell liposarcoma	t(12;16)(q13;p11)	*CHOP/TLS*
Pleomorphic liposarcoma	Increased chromosome numbers with complex rearrangements	

IC is of limited value. Widespread positive staining for desmin favours myxoid leiomyosarcoma. DNA ploidy analysis is also of limited value. An uniequivocal non-diploid cellular population is consistent with sarcoma.

If both the clinical history (rapidly growing, tender tumour) and the cytological features are typical, an attitude of 'wait and see' is justifiable since the vast majority of nodular fasciitis regress considerably or disappear within 4–5 weeks.

Desmoid Fibromatosis

Almost all cases needled are abdominal and extra-abdominal. In our experience the rare intra-abdominal fibromatoses are uncommon targets for FNA. Common sites for extra-abdominal desmoids are the proximal extremities and the shoulder and pelvic girdles.

Histopathology

Desmoid fibromatosis typically has poorly defined, infiltrative margins and is composed of bands or fascicles of fibroblasts with fusiform nuclei and elongated cytoplasm. Abundant collagen is present in the stroma and a myxoid matrix may be seen focally.

Cytological features of desmoid fibromatosis (fig. 28a–c)

Variable yield
Mixture of individual cells and cell clusters
Fragments of paucicellular collagenous stroma
Fibroblasts with spindle-shaped or fusiform nuclei, moderate anisokaryosis
Stripped nuclei
Preserved cells elongated with cytoplasmic processes

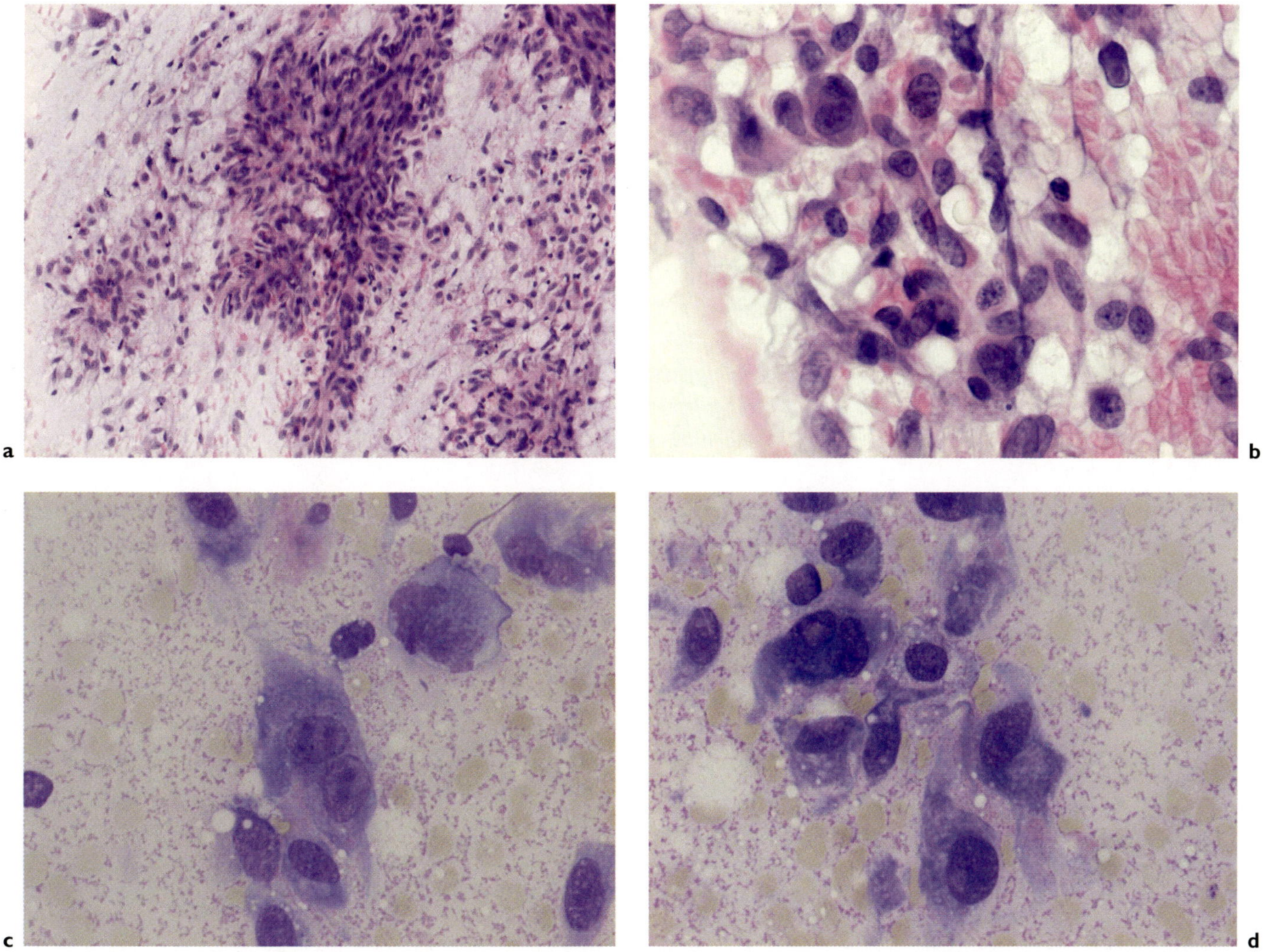

Fig. 26. Nodular fasciitis. **a** An abundant yield of both cell clusters and dispersed cells is characteristic of nodular fasciitis. The myxoid background matrix is only faintly visible in HE. Low magnification. **b** A pleomorphic population of (myo)fibroblasts is characteristic. HE. High magnification. **c**, **d** Binucleated ganglion cell-like cells are found in most smears. The myxoid background is evident. MGG. High magnification.

If infiltrating striated muscle, regenerating multinucleated muscle fibres ('muscle giant cells')

Differential diagnosis

Nodular fasciitis
Deep-seated leiomyoma
Low-grade fibrosarcoma
Low-grade malignant peripheral nerve sheath tumour (MPNST)
Monophasic fibrous synovial sarcoma

Comment

Abundant collagenous matrix may make needling difficult; the yield may be poor in spite of vigorous aspiration. If the yield is poor and does not include the characteristic mixture of collagen fragments and fibroblasts, differential diagnosis of the spindle cell tumours noted above is difficult. Smears of a desmoid with myxoid matrix may be mistaken for nodular fasciitis but the cell population of desmoids is less pleomorphic than that of nodular fasciitis, and the ganglion cell-like cells are not present. IC is of limited help; positive staining for S-100 protein or widespread desmin positivity excludes desmoid.

Solitary Fibrous Tumour

Solitary fibrous tumour may occur in almost any site of the body besides the pleura.

Those of soft tissue most often occur in adults as a deep-seated mass.

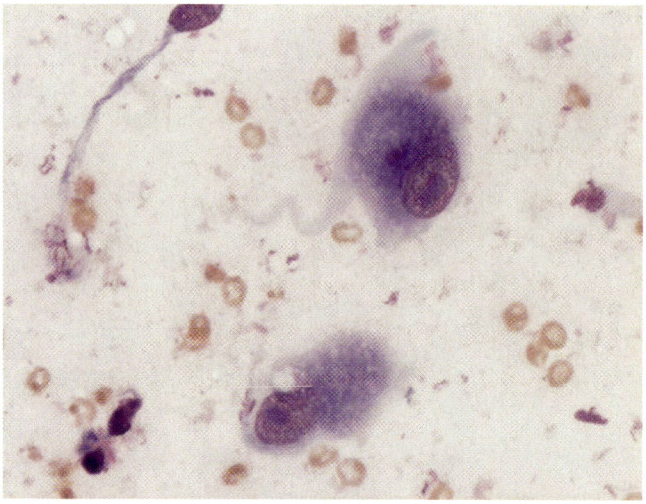

27

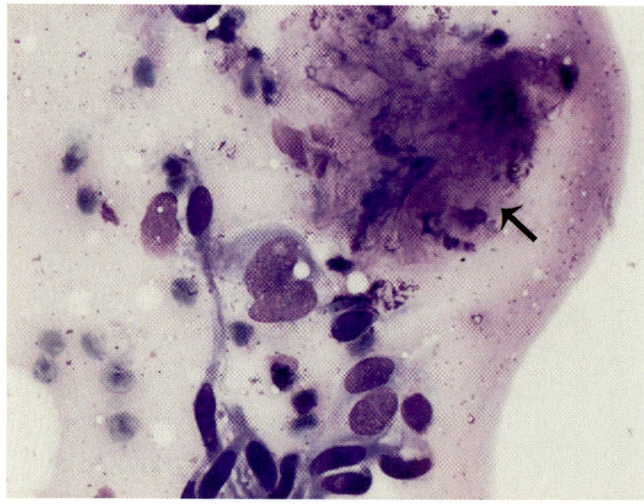

28a

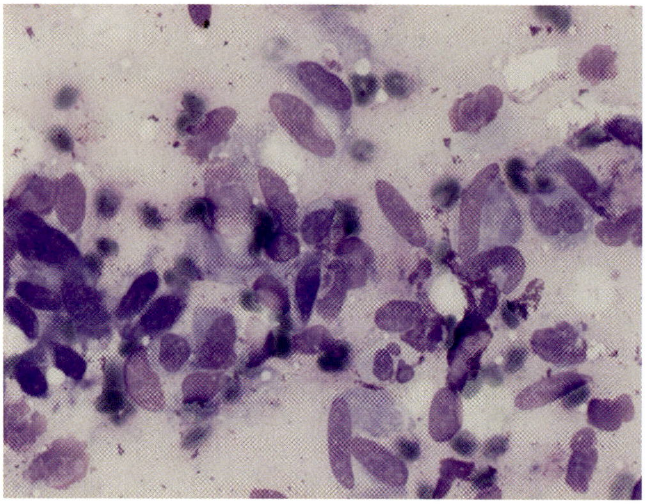

28b

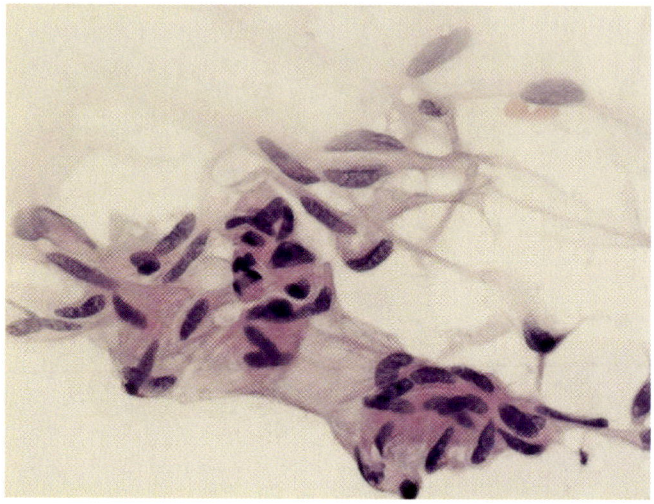

28c

Fig. 27. Proliferative myositis. Uni- or binucleated cells with abundant cytoplasm and large nuclei with prominent nucleoli predominate in proliferative myositis. MGG. High magnification.
Fig. 28. Desmoid fibromatosis. **a** A characteristic feature is the association of fibroblasts with collagenous stromal fragments (arrow). MGG. Medium magnification. **b**, **c** The cell population consists of fibroblasts with spindle-shaped or ovoid nuclei. A moderate anisokaryosis is not uncommon. MGG, HE. High magnification.

Histopathology

The main histological features are spindle cells arranged in a non-specific pattern, variable cellularity, thin bands of collagen between tumour cells, focal hyalinization, foci with a myxoid matrix, and a vascular pattern resembling haemangiopericytoma. The cells are fibroblast-like, almost always positive for CD34 and often for CD99 and bcl-2.

The cytological appearance of solitary fibrous tumour not related to the pleura has been described in a series of 8 cases [76].

Cytological features of solitary fibrous tumour (fig. 29a–d)

- Variable yield
- Dispersed cells mixed with cell-tight three-dimensional fascicle-like clusters
- Stripped nuclei between clusters
- Rather uniform population of spindle cells
- Nuclei with bland chromatin structure and inconspicuous nucleoli

Differential diagnosis

- Monophasic fibrous synovial sarcoma
- Low-grade fibrosarcoma
- Low-grade MPNST
- Malignant haemangiopericytoma

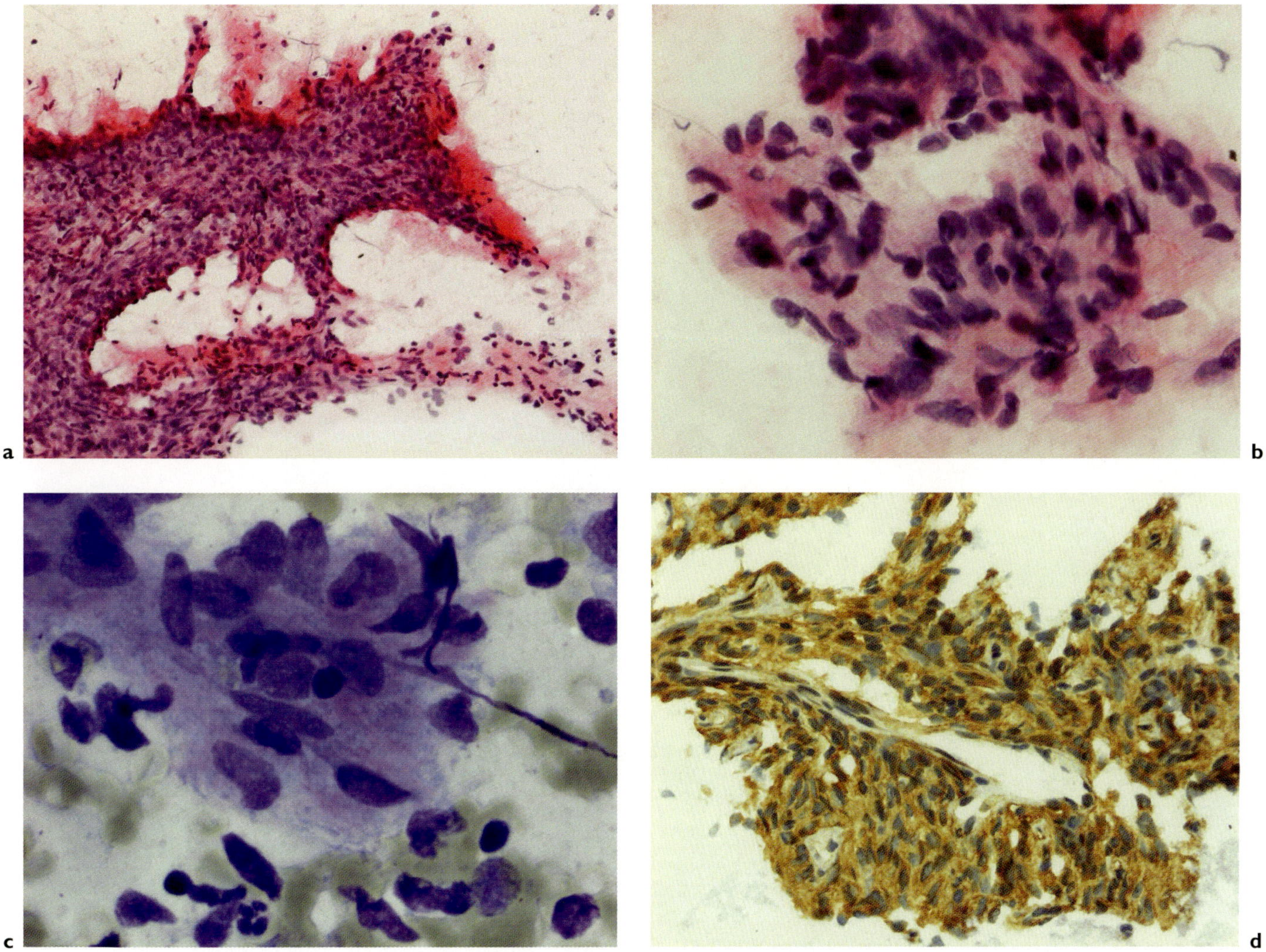

Fig. 29. Solitary fibrous tumour. **a** A cell-tight three-dimensional fragment surrounded by dispersed cells. HE. Low magnification. **b**, **c** The constituent cells are spindle-shaped with bland nuclei. HE and MGG. High magnification. **d** Positive CD34 staining. Cell block preparation. Medium magnification.

Comment

Cellular and nuclear atypia is usually more marked in fibrosarcoma and MPNST than in solitary fibrous tumour. A correct diagnosis of solitary fibrous tumour is, however, difficult on routinely stained material. IC is of diagnostic help. If the spindle cell population is positive for CD34, CD99 and bcl-2, fibrosarcoma, MPNST and synovial sarcoma are all excluded.

Elastofibroma

Elastofibroma is typically a slowly growing mass beneath the scapula in elderly females.

Histopathology

Elastofibroma is composed of (myo)fibroblasts. Its characteristic feature is faulty elastin fibrillogenesis. Tissue sections show a hypocellular, collagenous lesion containing numerous eosinophilic elastic fibres, either in rounded aggregates or as serrated fibres.

The cytological appearance in FNA smears has been described in individual case reports [77, 78].

Cytological features of elastofibroma (fig. 30a–d)

Variable yield, often hypocellular smears

Variable amount of spindly, fibroblast-like cells, singly or in loosely cohesive groups

Variable amount of fragments of elastic fibres, typically serrated

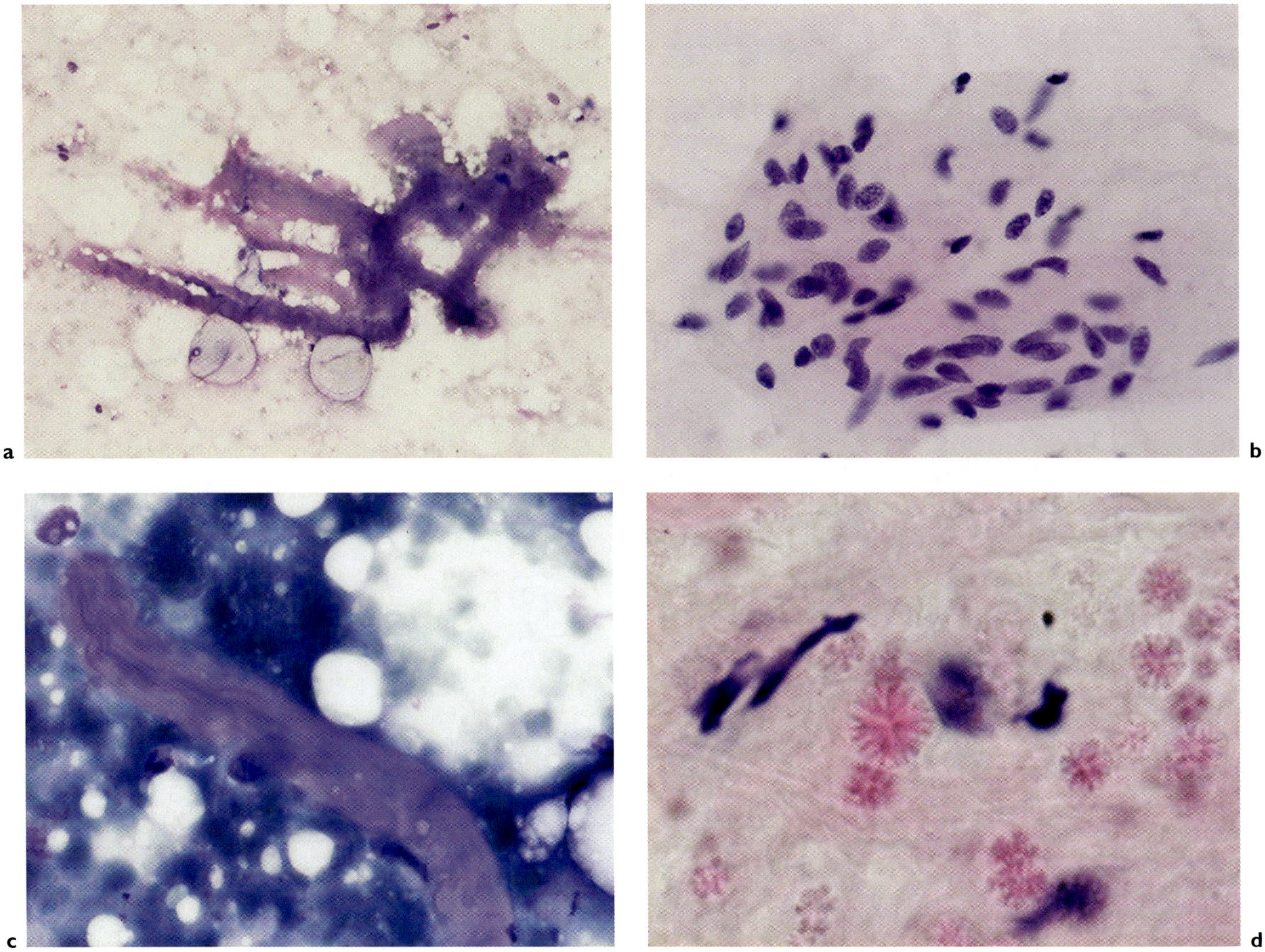

Fig. 30. Elastofibroma. **a** A hypocellular smear of spindly, fibroblast-like cells, dominated by elastic fibres. MGG. Low magnification. **b** The fibroblast-like cells have uniform bland nuclei. HE. Medium magnification. **c**, **d** The diagnostic feature of elastofibroma is the presence of fragments of serrated elastic fibres. MGG, at times appearing in the smears as cog-wheel-like structures. HE. High magnification.

Comment

The cytological diagnosis of elastofibroma is difficult. The main diagnostic feature is the presence of degenerate elastic fibres.

Malignant Tumours

Adult Fibrosarcoma

Adult fibrosarcoma is at present considered as a rare tumour and a diagnosis of exclusion. It is a deep-seated tumour of elderly adults and the limbs are the most frequent sites. The majority of sarcomas formerly diagnosed as fibrosarcoma are today classified either as monophasic synovial sarcoma or MPNST.

Histopathology

The pattern is fascicular, the fascicles of cells are often arranged in a herringbone-like pattern. The tumour cells are fibroblast-like, exhibiting variable nuclear atypia. The stroma is variably fibrous.

Cytological features of adult fibrosarcoma

- Uniform population of spindle cells, both dispersed and arranged in clusters or fascicular structures
- Stripped nuclei not uncommon
- Spindle-shaped cells with fusiform nuclei and elongated cytoplasm

Variable cellular and nuclear atypia (high-grade malignant tumours have hyperchromatic nuclei with coarse chromatin and prominent nucleoli)

Differential diagnosis

Desmoid
Solitary fibrous tumour
Monophasic fibrous synovial sarcoma
MPNST

Comment

Adult fibrosarcoma is most often diagnosed as a spindle cell sarcoma, not otherwise specified. IC is of limited help. Adult fibrosarcoma may express muscle actin and desmin. CD34 and S-100 protein are usually negative.

Low-Grade Fibromyxoid Sarcoma

Low-grade fibromyxoid sarcoma, described by Evans [79] and Goodlad et al. [80] in series of cases, is clinically as well as morphologically considered to be a specific entity separate from low-grade myxofibrosarcoma.

Histopathology

Bland, uniform spindle cells, often arranged in a whorled pattern, are seen within a variably myxoid and variably collagenous stroma. The border between myxoid and collagenous areas is often sharp. Vascularity is generally low but curvolinear vessels are present in myxoid areas. Mitotic activity is low. Immunohistochemically only vimentin stains positively in most cases. Focal staining for CD34 and actin has been reported.

The cytological profile has been described in one case report [81]. The features were similar to the individual cases in our files.

Cytological features of low-grade fibromyxoid sarcoma (fig. 31a–c)

Abundant myxoid background
Dispersed cells and cell clusters
Often stripped nuclei
Homogenous population of fibroblast-like spindle-shaped cells with mildly atypical nuclei
Poor vascularity, almost no vessel fragments seen in the background

Differential diagnosis

Intramuscular myxoma
Perineurioma
Low-grade myxofibrosarcoma

Comment

Low-grade fibromyxoid sarcoma is most often misdiagnosed as a low-grade myxofibrosarcoma due to the myxoid background and the atypical spindle cells. From the clinical point of view this is not a serious mistake as the treatment (primary surgery) is the same for both sarcomas. Intramuscular myxoma is usually less cellular in FNA smears than fibromyxoid sarcoma. IC is helpful in the differential diagnosis against perineurioma, which stains positively for EMA.

Fibrous Tumours in Infancy and Childhood

Of the various fibrous tumours/lesions in infancy and childhood, fibromatosis colli (torticollis) is often subjected to FNA, fibrous hamartoma of infancy and infantile fibrosarcoma rarely.

Benign Tumours

Fibromatosis Colli (Torticollis)

Fibromatosis colli presents itself as a firm tumour-like mass in the side of the neck (within the sternocleidomastoid muscle) in newborn infants.

Histopathology

There is a diffuse proliferation of fibroblasts within the muscle. The involved muscle fibres are atrophic and have multiple nuclei resembling large multinucleated giant cells. The cytological appearances of fibromatosis colli have been presented in one large series [82] together with case reports.

Cytological features of fibromatosis colli (fig. 32a, b)

Tufts of myxoid matrix in the background
Mixture of dispersed and clustered bland-looking fibroblast-like cells
Many stripped nuclei
More or less numerous, most often multinucleated regenerating muscle fibres ('muscle giant cells')

Differential diagnosis

Pleomorphic sarcoma

Comment

The double population of spindle cells and muscle giant cells is typical. The muscle giant cells have an abundant eosinophilic (wet fixed smears) or deep-blue (MGG) cytoplasm containing rows of uniform rounded nuclei with prominent nucleoli. Uninuclear tadpole-shaped muscle cells may be seen.

Many cases regress spontaneously and the primary therapy is conservative.

a 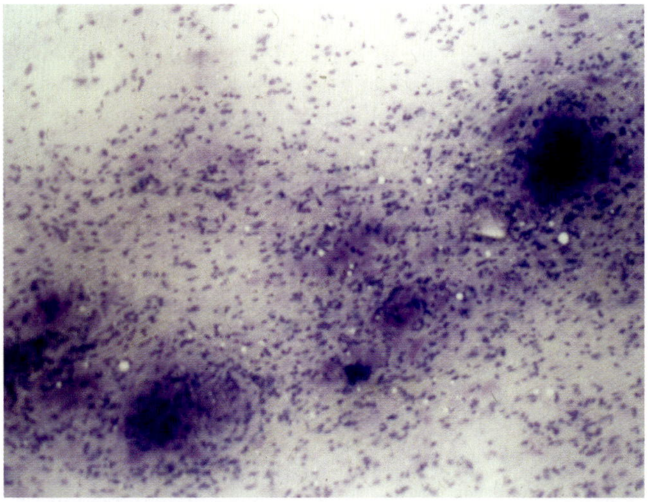

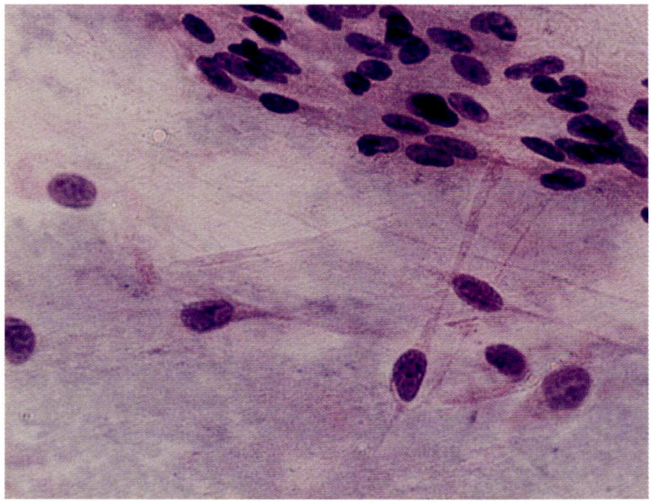 b

c 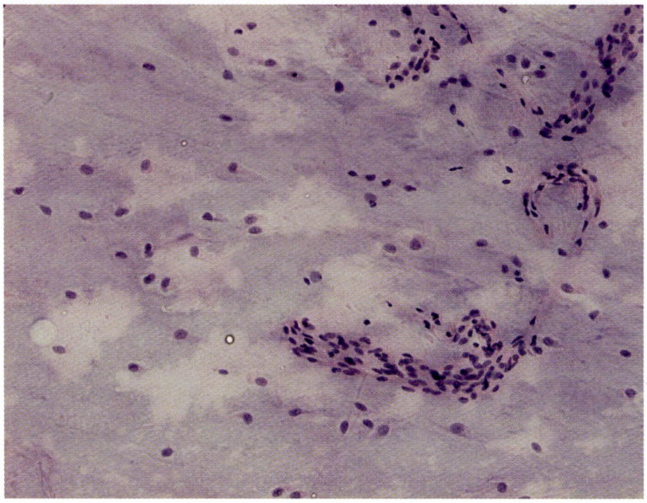

Fig. 31. Low-grade fibromyxoid sarcoma. **a** Dispersed cells and tight cell clusters in an abundant myxoid background substance. MGG. Low magnification. **b** Uniform population of mildly atypical fibroblast-like cells. MGG. High magnification. **c** Curved vessel fragments may be seen in the myxoid background. When vessel fragments are present it is not possible to distinguish between low-grade fibromyxoid sarcoma and low-grade myxofibrosarcoma in FNA smears. HE. Low magnification.

Fibrous Hamartoma of Infancy

Fibrous hamartoma of infancy is very rare after the age of 2 years and typically presents as a subcutaneous mass in the upper arm or around the shoulder.

Histopathology

This lesion has ill-defined boundaries and is composed of a mixture of mature adipose tissue, fibrous septa or bands and myxoid foci with small rounded primitive cells.

The features of fibrous hamartoma of infancy have been described in individual case reports [83].

Cytological features of fibrous hamartoma of infancy (fig. 33a, b)

Mixture of mature adipose tissue and clusters or runs of spindly cells

More or less abundant tufts of myxoid background substance

The spindle cells are uniform with bland nuclei

Differential diagnosis

Infantile fibrosarcoma

Malignant Tumours

Infantile Fibrosarcoma

Infantile fibrosarcoma may be congenital and is generally seen before the age of 2. Most infantile fibrosarcomas arise in the arms or legs and present as a large, non-tender mass.

Histopathology

Fascicles of tightly packed fibroblasts with slight nuclear atypia and often numerous mitoses. Myxoid stroma and areas of round cells as well as a haemangiopericytoma-like vascular pattern may be seen. Lymphocytic infiltrates and haemorrhages and foci of necrosis may be found.

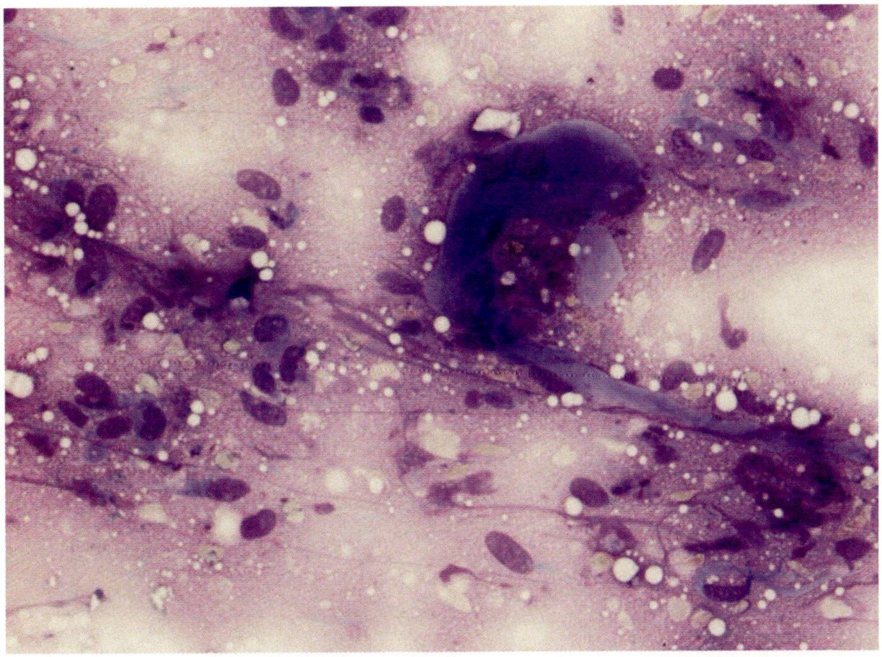

a

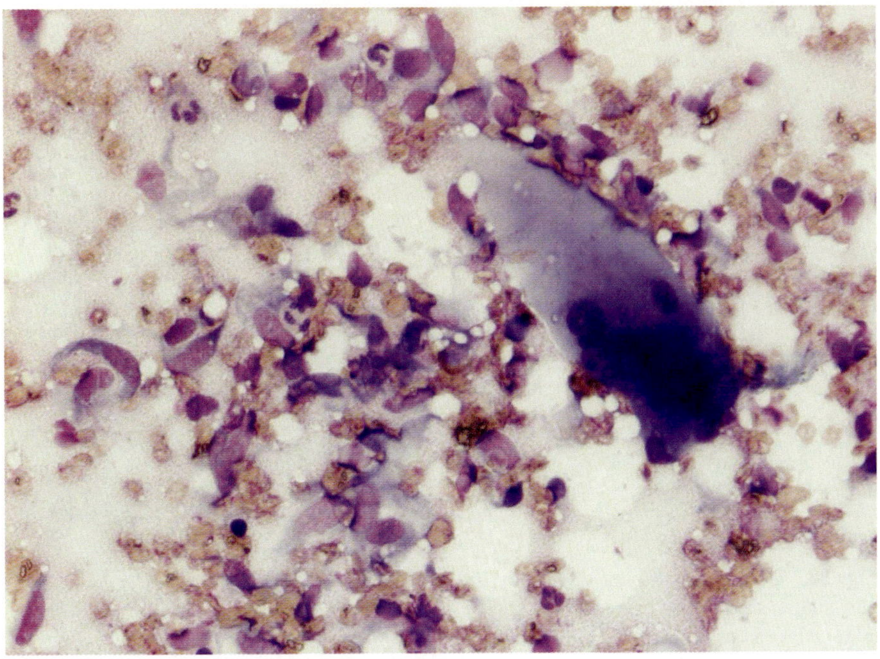

b

Fig. 32. Fibromatosis colli. **a** All the features characteristic of fibromatosis colli are present in this field: myxoid background, bland-looking fibroblast-like cells and 'muscle giant cells'. MGG. Low magnification. **b** The 'muscle giant cells' are often a prominent feature. MGG. High magnification.

Infantile fibrosarcoma is rarely described in the cytological literature. We have needled one case, a large tumour in the lower leg.

Cytological features of infantile fibrosarcoma (fig. 34a, b)

Rich yield

Clusters, runs or fascicular fragments of three-dimensional tightly packed spindle cells

The cellular population is uniform, nuclei bland with slight atypia

Mitoses

Differential diagnosis

Embryonal rhabdomyosarcoma

Childhood fibromatosis

Fibrous hamartoma of infancy

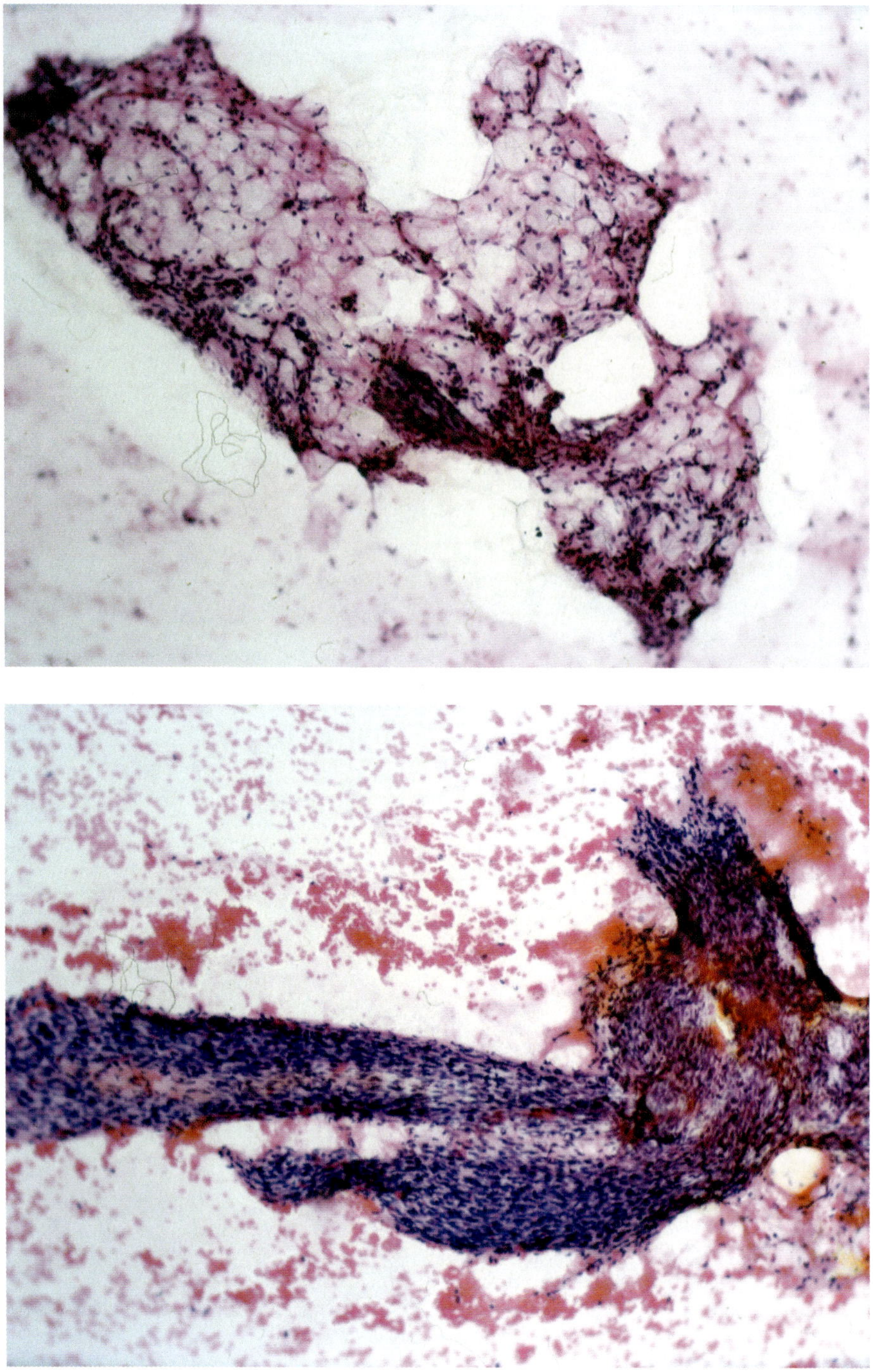

a

b

Fig. 33. Fibrous hamartoma of infancy. In our single case there were fragments of mature fat (**a**) as well as three-dimensional cell-tight fascicles of spindle cells (**b**). HE. Low magnification.

Comment

In our limited experience the spindle cell population is very similar in FNA smears of fibrous hamartoma and of infantile fibrosarcoma. Infantile fibrosarcoma showing a mixture of round and spindle cells may be mistaken for rhabdomyosarcoma. IC and EM are helpful in this differential diagnosis.

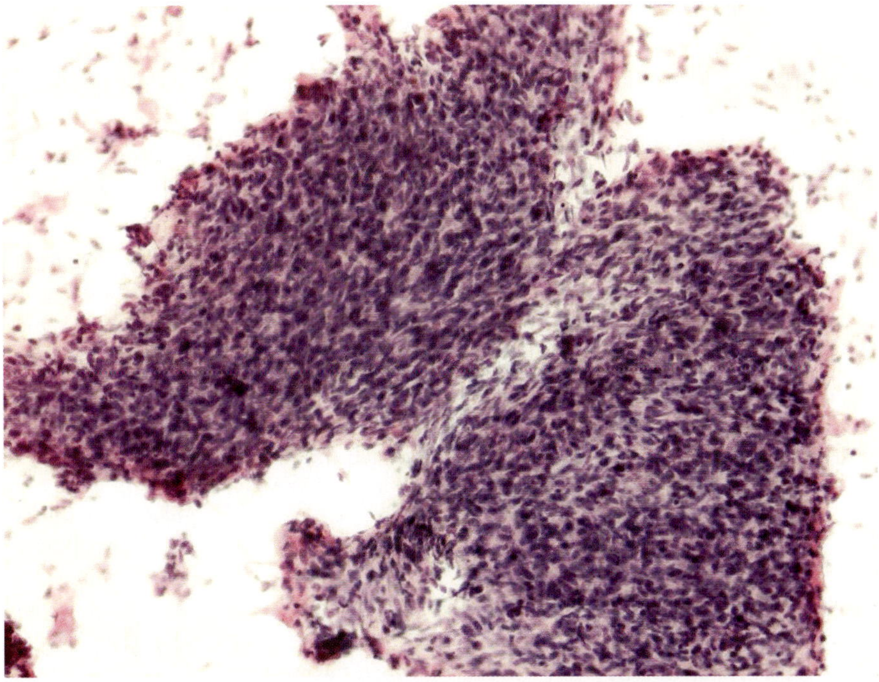

a

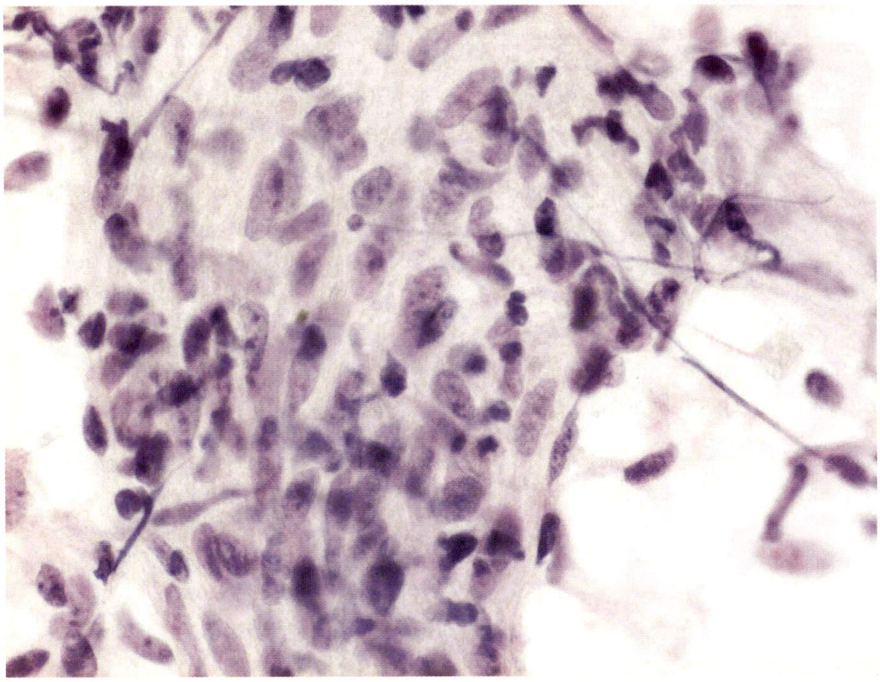

b

Fig. 34. Infantile fibrosarcoma. **a** In our only case there was an abundant yield of three-dimensional fascicular fragments composed of tightly packed spindle cells. HE. Low magnification. **b** The cell population is uniform and has bland, slightly atypical spindly nuclei. HE. High magnification.

Fibrohistiocytic Tumours

Some of the variants of fibrohistiocytic tumours are the most common objects of FNA. Myxofibrosarcoma and 'malignant fibrous histiocytoma' are the most frequent sarcomas referred for FNA, localized giant cell tumour of tendon sheath is part of the soft tissue tumour spectrum in every FNA clinic and some cases of dermatofibrosarcoma protuberans are also biopsied.

Benign Tumours

Localized Tumour of Tendon Sheath

This is a common tumour of the digits, presenting as a painless, slowly growing nodule usually 1–3 cm in diameter at the time of FNA biopsy.

Histopathology

The tumour is composed of rounded mononuclear cells, osteoclast-like giant cells, xanthoma cells, siderophages and inflammatory cells in variable proportions. The stroma may be hyalinized in some tumours, and cellular examples may exhibit numerous mitoses.

The cytological features in FNA smears match the histological pattern fairly well.

Cytological features of localized tumour of tendon sheath (fig. 35a–c)

- Variable yield; lesions with extensive hyalinization are poor in cells
- Mononuclear, rounded cells with rounded vesicular nuclei, dispersed and in clusters
- Moderate anisocytosis and anisokaryosis common
- Variable presence of multinucleated osteoclast-like giant cells
- Variable presence of histiocytes (with foamy, vacuolated cytoplasm and/or haemosiderin laden)
- Mitoses may be present

Comment

The clinical presentation and the cytological features are indicative of this diagnosis.

Malignant Tumours

Dermatofibrosarcoma protuberans

Dermatofibrosarcoma protuberans is most commonly seen in adults, often with a long, 5 years or more, history of a slowly growing dermal/subcutaneous tumour. Tumours referred for FNA are almost exclusively exophytic-nodular.

Histopathology

The most characteristic pattern is that of relatively bland spindle cells with elongated nuclei arranged in a storiform pattern. The typical immunohistochemical profile is a double positivity for vimentin and CD34. The cytological features have been described in two series [53, 54].

Cytological features of dermatofibrosarcoma protuberans (fig. 36a–d)

- Uniform population of spindle cells, dispersed, clustered or in three-dimensional cell-rich fascicles (fascicular arrangement)
- Moderate variation in nuclear size and shape, bland nuclear chromatin, small nucleoli
- Occasionally adipose tissue fragments infiltrated by runs of spindle cells

Differential diagnosis

- Cellular fibrous histiocytoma
- Other spindle cell sarcomas located in the cutis-subcutis

Comment

Cellular smears from dermatofibrosarcoma protuberans are most often considered as low-grade malignant spindle cell sarcoma. The most important differential diagnosis is cellular benign fibrous histiocytoma. The presence of histiocytes and/or giant cells favours histiocytoma. Furthermore, the spindle cells in fibrous histiocytoma are CD34 negative.

Malignant Fibrous Histiocytoma

Since MFH was recognized as a specific sarcoma entity in 1963, it has almost universally been regarded as the most common soft tissue sarcoma. However, during the last 10 years the concept of MFH as a specific entity has been questioned because of the obvious clinical and morphological heterogeneity among the various subtypes, storiform/pleomorphic, myxoid, giant cell, angiomatoid and inflammatory. Because of this clinical and morphological heterogeneity, it has been suggested that MFH may represent an anaplastic variant of a number of other soft tissue sarcomas with a specific line of differentiation. In retrospective evaluations of sarcomas primarily diagnosed as MFH, especially the storiform/pleomorphic variant, it has been shown that myogenic, lipogenic and Schwann cell differentiation has been present in parts of the tumours in question [84, 85]. Angiomatoid as well as myxoid MFH have been regarded as specific entities [86].

Due to these current opinions we avoid the diagnosis of MFH in FNA material. We suggest descriptive diagnoses such as pleomorphic sarcoma or high-grade malignant spindle cell/pleomorphic sarcoma unless a specific line of differentiation can be proved by the combined evaluation of routine stains and ancillary methods. Pleomorphic sarcoma of the 'MFH type' has been microscopically evaluated in FNA samples in two large series [26, 27].

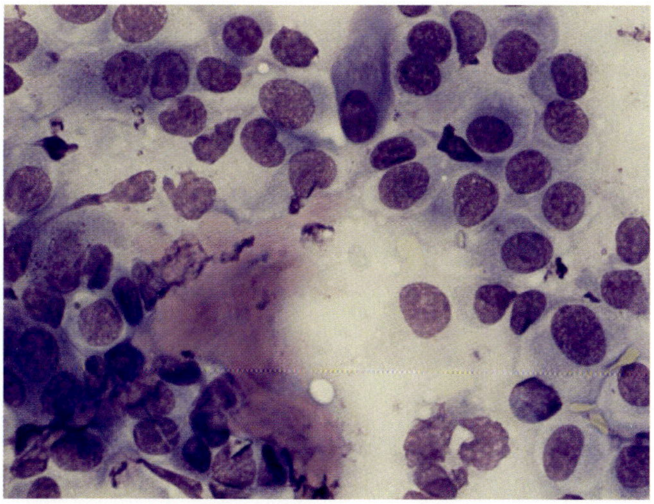

a

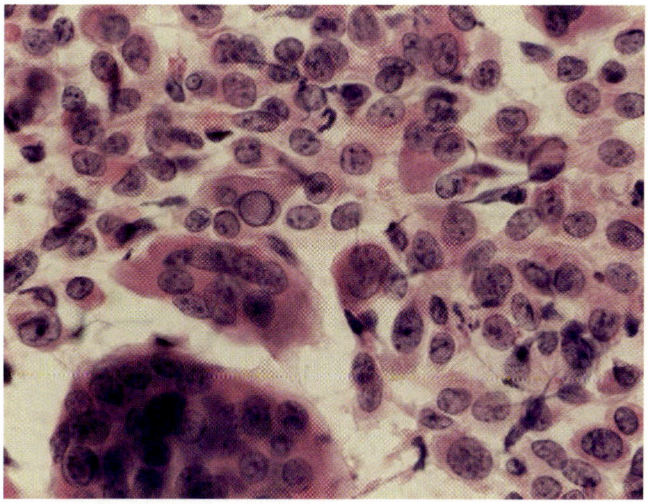

b

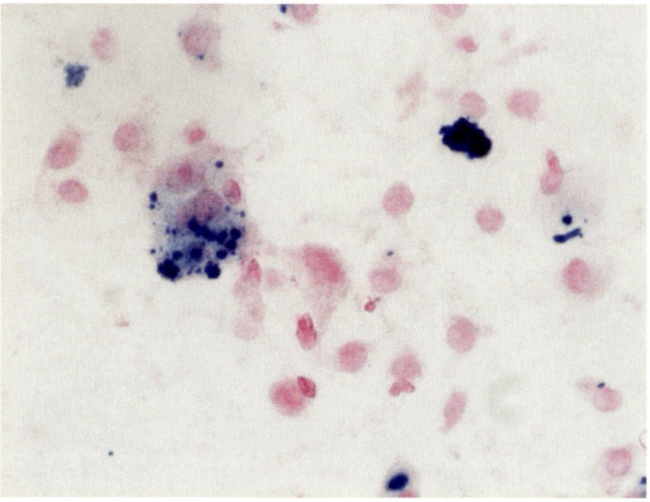

c

Fig. 35. Localized tumour of tendon sheath. **a** Mononuclear, rounded tumour cells with rounded nuclei. Mild anisokaryosis is common. MGG. High magnification. **b** More or less numerous multinucleated osteoclast-like giant cells are always present in the smears. HE. High magnification. **c** An iron stain (Prussian blue) highlights the haemosiderin-laden histiocytes. Prussian blue. High magnification.

Cytological features of malignant fibrous histiocytoma (fig. 37a–c)

- Often highly cellular smears
- Necrosis, cystic degeneration and haemorrhage often present
- Tissue fragments, cell clusters and dispersed cells in varying proportions
- Variable proportions of atypical spindle cells, rounded or polygonal cells with abundant cytoplasm, and multinucleated large cells
- Generally marked nuclear pleomorphism, irregular coarse chromatin and prominent nucleoli
- Mitotic figures, including atypical

Differential diagnosis

- Soft tissue metastasis from anaplastic large cell carcinoma
- Soft tissue metastasis from sarcomatous melanoma
- Soft tissue presentation of ALCL (sarcomatous giant cell variant)

Comment

Anaplastic carcinoma, malignant melanoma as well as ALCL may present the same pleomorphism, including a mixture of atypical spindle cells and multinucleated giant cells, as in pleomorphic sarcoma. Cytological features indicating epithelial differentiation are small moulded groups of tumour cells looking like 'owls' eyes'. The cellular population in ALCL, although pleomorphic, is predominantly made up of rounded cells with dark blue cytoplasm (MGG) with the presence of Reed-Sternberg-like cells. One exception is the sarcomatous variant of ALCL. Immunocytochemistry is the best ancillary method to apply in the differential diagnosis. The lymphoma cells are always strongly positive for CD30 and in the majority of cases for EMA. According to the literature up to 80% of ALCL are ALK positive as well. Cytokeratins, HMB45 and Melan A, are other useful antibodies in the differential diagnosis.

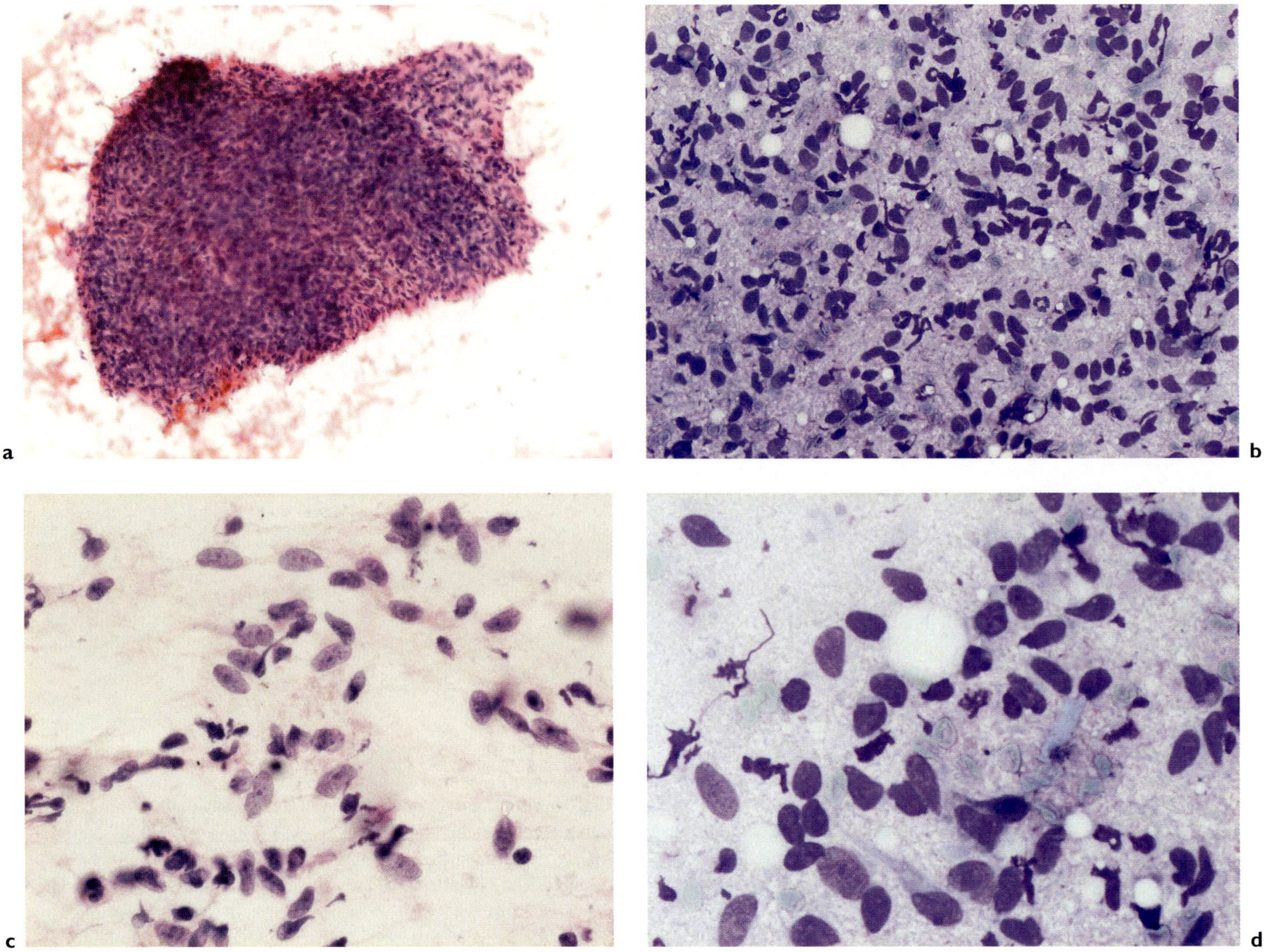

Fig. 36. Dermatofibrosarcoma protuberans. **a** Spindle cells forming three-dimensional, cell-tight fascicles. HE. Low magnification. **b** Stripped nuclei and a cytoplasmic background substance are often present. MGG. Low magnification. **c, d** The tumour cells exhibit mild pleomorphism, bland nuclear chromatin and small nucleoli. HE, MGG. High magnification.

Myxofibrosarcoma (Myxoid Type of MFH)

The typical clinical presentation of myxofibrosarcoma is that of a subcutaneous tumour. Myxofibrosarcoma occurs most commonly in the limbs of elderly patients (60–80 years of age) [86].

Histopathology

Low-grade malignant tumours are predominantly composed of slightly atypical spindle and stellate cells while high-grade sarcomas are pleomorphic showing marked cellular atypia and multinucleated tumour cells. Irrespective of the malignancy grade, numerous thin-walled curvolinear vessels are present in the myxoid background in fewer cellular areas. Tumour cells with vacuolated cytoplasm are also found (pseudolipoblasts).

The appearance of myxofibrosarcoma in smears has been reported in two series [28, 29].

Cytological features of myxofibrosarcoma (fig. 38a–e)

Abundant myxoid background; macroscopically aspirates often appear as droplets of haemorrhagic glue-like fluid

Dispersed cells, small cell clusters and cellular aggregates

In low-grade tumours predominantly mildly atypical spindle cells with a few scattered large rounded polygonal cells

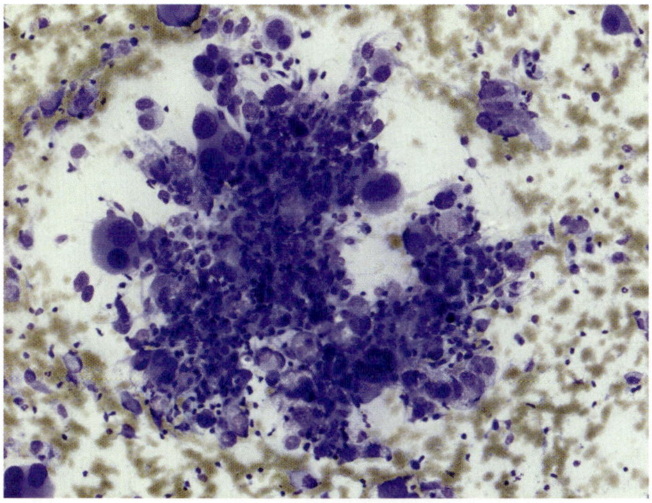

a

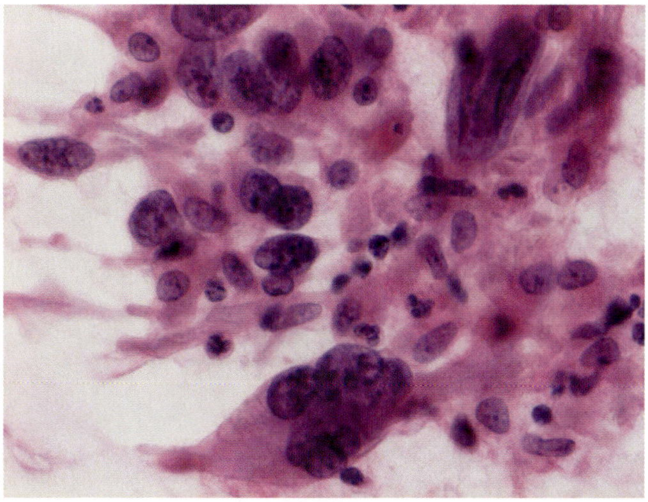

b

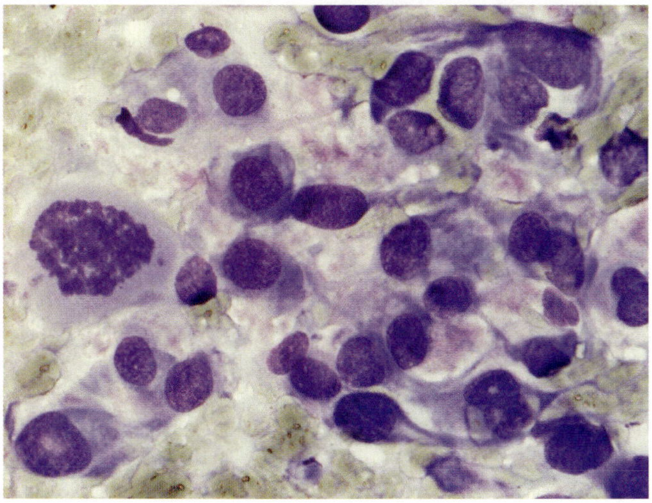

c

Fig. 37. 'Malignant fibrous histiocytoma'. **a** A cellular cluster of pleomorphic tumour cells. Note the marked variation in cell size. MGG. Low magnification. **b** Typical pleomorphic appearance in a smear of a 'malignant fibrous histiocytoma'. HE. High magnification. **c** Mitotic figures are a common finding in high-grade malignant tumours. MGG. High magnification.

Some cells have a vacuolated cytoplasm or contain droplets of mucoid material (blue-violet in MGG)
Marked nuclear pleomorphism in high-grade tumours
Fragments of curved vessels present in the myxoid background; few vessels in relation to cell clusters or aggregates

Differential diagnosis
Intramuscular myxoma
Nodular fasciitis
Myxoid liposarcoma
Low-grade fibromyxoid sarcoma

Comment

The distinction between nodular fasciitis, intramuscular myxoma and low-grade myxofibrosarcoma is most important from the clinical point of view. The vascular architecture is one discriminating cytological feature. In myxoma and in nodular fasciitis, no or only individual fragments of coarse vessels are found in the myxoid background, while myxofibrosarcoma frequently exhibits curved coarser vessel fragments best observed in pancicellular areas.

IC is of limited value. S-100 protein positivity in lipoblast-like cells is a feature of myxoid liposarcoma.

The tumour cells in myxofibrosarcoma are focally actin positive and consistently vimentin positive.

Smooth Muscle Tumours

Benign smooth muscle tumours are infrequently needled. Cutaneous leiomyoma as well as angioleiomyoma are, in our experience, seldom referred for FNA.

The very uncommon deep leiomyoma of soft tissue, however, is biopsied occasionally.

a
b
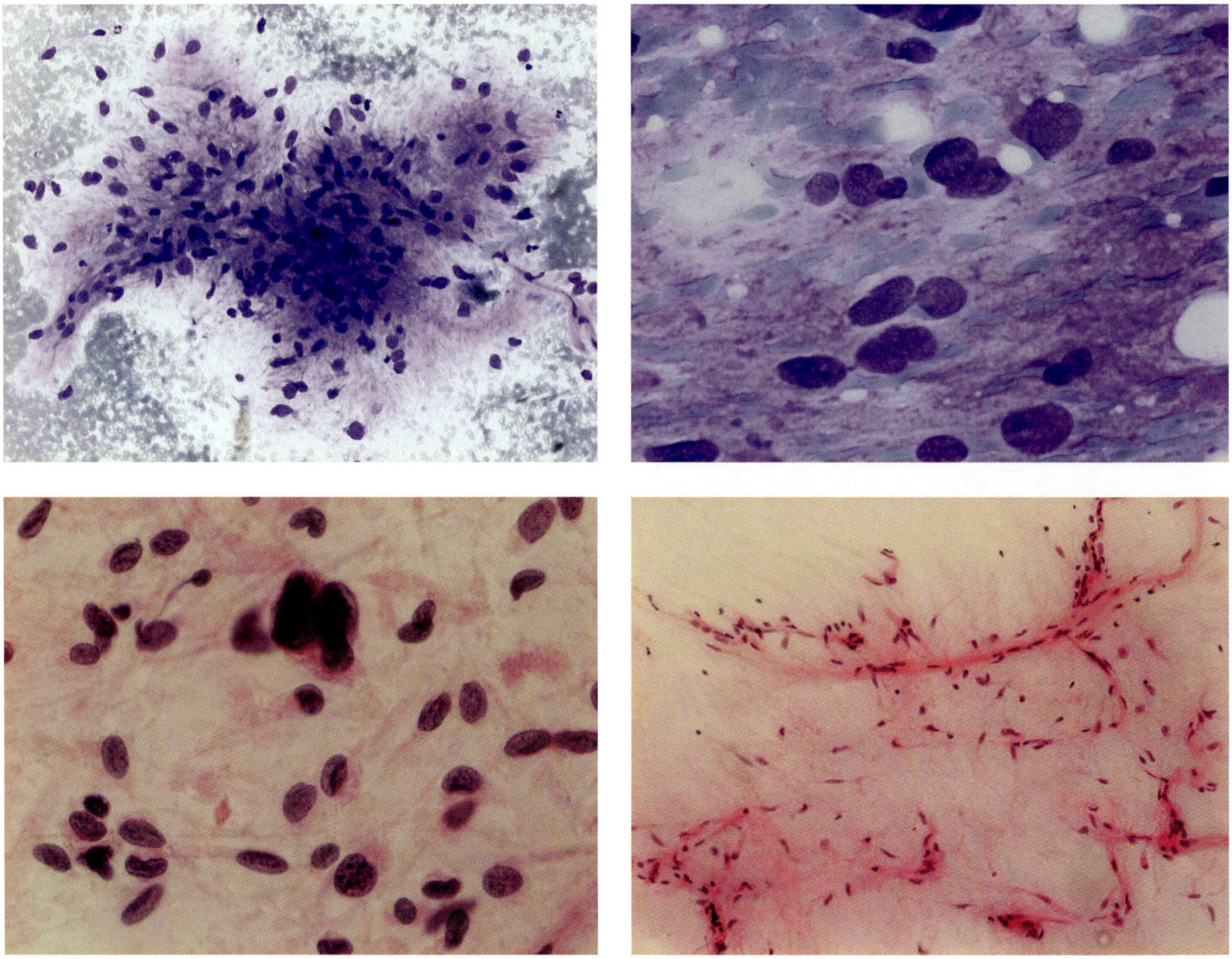
c
d
e
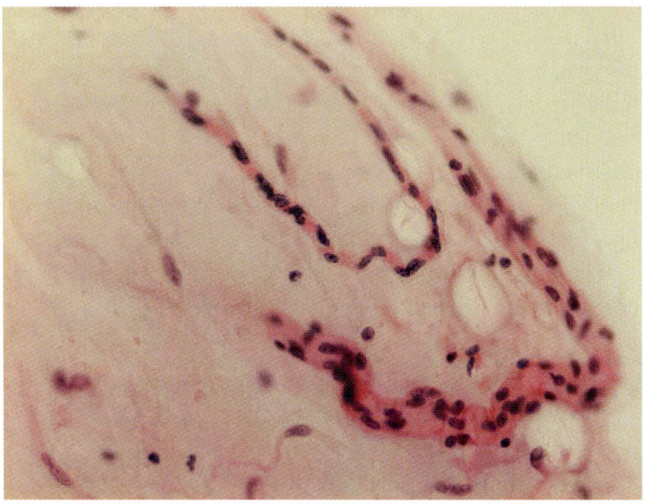

Fig. 38. Myxofibrosarcoma, low and high grade. **a** Cell clusters and dispersed cells in a myxoid background. MGG. Low magnification. **b** Mildly atypical spindle cells from a low-grade tumour. MGG. High magnification. **c** Cellular atypia is obvious in this high-grade tumour. HE. High magnification. **d**, **e** Irrespective of grade, curved vessel fragments in the myxoid background are an important diagnostic sign. HE. High magnification.

Leiomyosarcoma is one of the most frequent sarcomas referred for FNA.

Benign Tumours

Deep Leiomyoma of Soft Tissue

This rare tumour is most common in the limbs and trunk. It is a slow-growing, well-circumscribed tumour, often 5 cm or more at diagnosis.

Histopathology

Deep leiomyomas are usually well-demarcated tumours with a lobular pattern. They are composed of typical smooth muscle cells. Hyalinization and a focally myxoid matrix are not uncommon. Deep leiomyomas are difficult to differentiate from low-grade leiomyosarcomas.

It has been stressed that tissue sections must be thoroughly investigated for mitotic figures; a diagnosis of deep leiomyoma is considered incorrect even if individual mitotic figures are found [87].

There are FNA smears from 5 cases of deep leiomyoma in our material.

Cytological features of deep leiomyoma (fig. 39a, b)

Clusters of loosely attached cells, small aggregates and dispersed cells
A bluish-red background matrix (MGG) is often seen in aggregates
Elongated nuclei; presence of blunt-ended, cigar-shaped and truncated nuclei
Finely granular chromatin and small nucleoli
Preserved, dispersed cells have elongated grey or blue cytoplasm (MGG)
Moderate anisocytosis and anisokaryosis
No mitotic figures

Differential diagnosis

Extra-abdominal desmoid
Low-grade leiomyosarcoma
Low-grade MPNST
Monophasic fibrous synovial sarcoma

Comment

Under low power the smear patterns of desmoid and leiomyoma are remarkably alike but the collagenous stromal fragments with degenerate nuclei, typical for desmoid, are not present in leiomyoma, and typical smooth muscle cell nuclei are not seen in desmoid. Smears from synovial sarcoma are generally more cellular with larger, more cellular aggregates, a more uniform cell population, and the presence of mitoses. Cigar-shaped and/or truncated nuclei are not present. Low-grade leiomyosarcoma is the most important diagnostic pitfall. Generally the tumour cells in leiomyosarcoma have a coarser chromatin structure. The presence of even a single mitosis should discourage the cytopathologist to diagnose a deep leiomyoma.

IC is of help in the differential diagnosis. A positive reaction with desmin or caldesmon or widespread positivity with SMA indicates that the tumour is of smooth muscle origin.

Angiomyoma (Angioleiomyoma)

Angiomyoma is a subcutaneous tumour usually on the limbs of middle-aged adults. It is typically a small tumour (up to 2 cm), distinctly tender at palpation and painful at aspiration. Angiomyomas are composed of smooth muscle cells and thick-walled vessels.

Histopathology

Angiomyomas are well-circumscribed tumours composed of cells resembling smooth muscle cells. The cells are intimately connected with smooth muscle cells of the thick-walled vessels, which are part of the tumour. The cells may show moderate pleomorphism. Only one study on the cytological appearance of angiomyoma in FNA material has been published [25].

Cytological features of angiomyoma (fig. 40a, b)

Moderate to poor yield
Predominantly dissociated cells, small sheets occasionally present
Spindle-shaped cells, some with features of smooth muscle cells
Rather uniform cells with finely dispersed nuclear chromatin and occasionally small nucleoli
Fragments of collagenous matrix with embedded spindle cells occasionally present
Fat cells infrequently included with the spindle cell population; presence of macrophages

Differential diagnosis

Nodular fasciitis
Neurilemoma
Fibrous histiocytoma
Granular cell tumour
Glomus tumour
Cutaneous cylindroma
Melanoma (spindle cell type)

Comment

None of the 10 cases in the published study [25] were correctly diagnosed. From a clinical point of view it is important

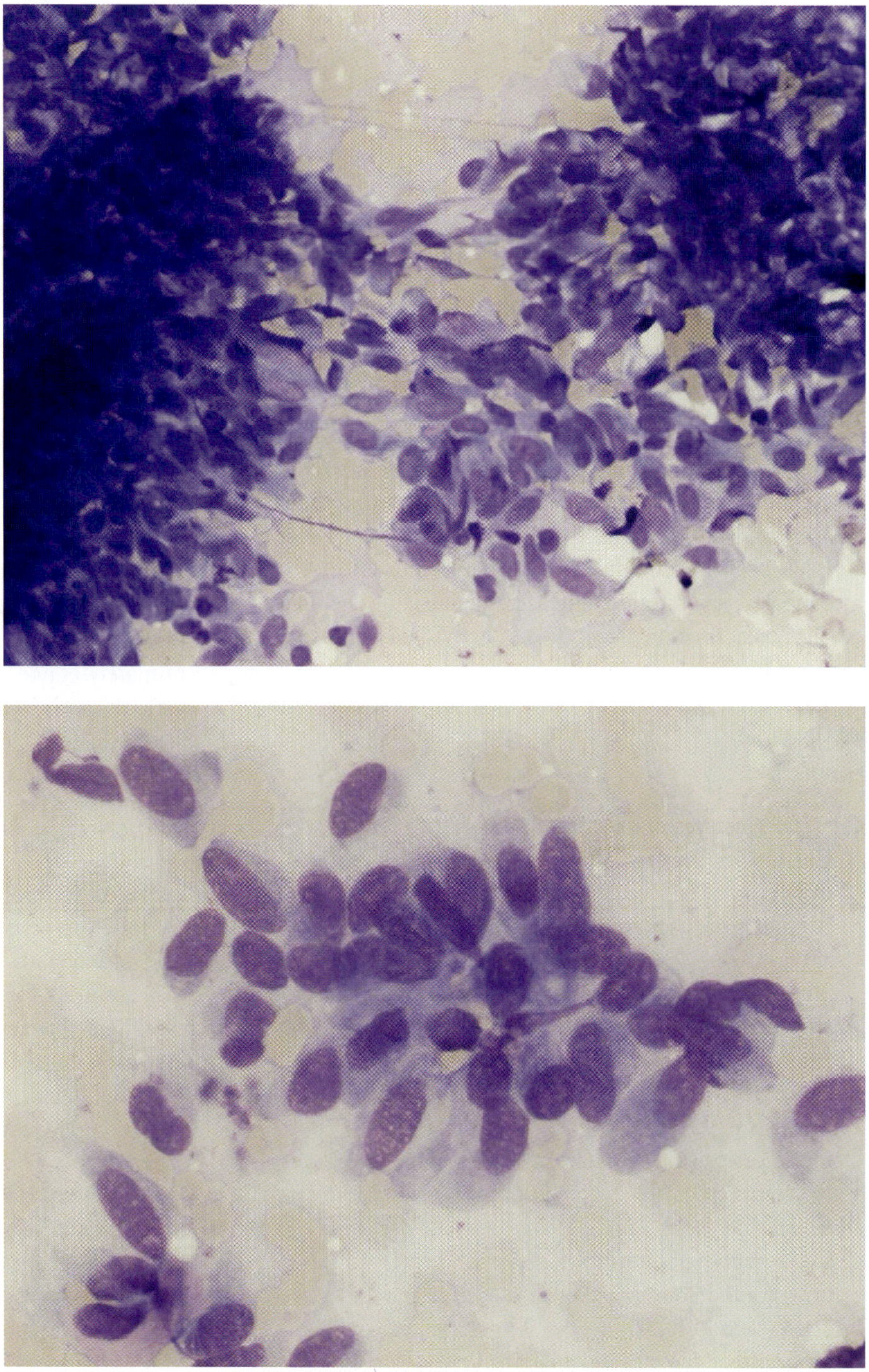

a

b

Fig. 39. Deep leiomyoma. **a** A cluster of loosely cohesive tumour cells with blunt-ended, benign-looking nuclei, and elongated grey-blue cytoplasm. MGG. Low magnification. **b** The uniform cigar-shaped nuclei and the grey-blue cytoplasm are evident in higher magnification. MGG. Intermediate magnification.

that the cytopathologist correctly diagnoses an angiomyoma as a benign tumour and excludes nodular fasciitis since most cases of nodular fasciitis regress and therefore only a wait-and-see strategy is adopted. As regards the other benign entities in the differential diagnoses, surgical intervention, if any, is the same. If smears are cellular or moderately cellular it is possible to exclude granular cell tumour and cutaneous cylindroma, as the cellular features of these lesions are not present in angiomyoma. Glomus tumours typically are subungual and composed of rounded cells. Neurilemoma is the most difficult pitfall as neurilemoma as well as angiomyoma are painful at needling and the cellular composition of the two entities is similar. If material can be saved for IC, staining for desmin and S-100 is helpful.

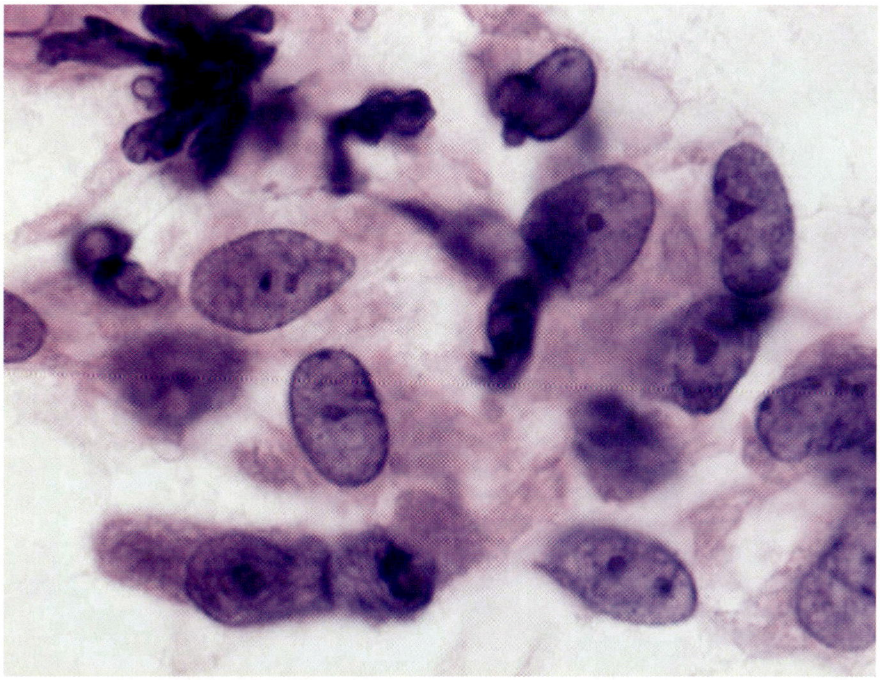

a

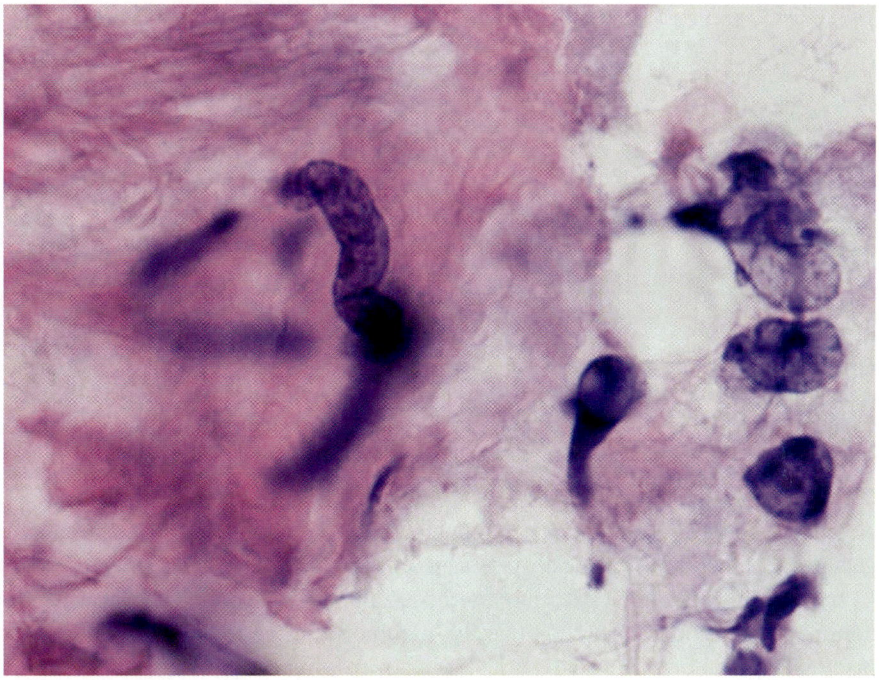

b

Fig. 40. Angiomyoma. **a** A small group of loosely cohesive uniform spindle-shaped cells with mostly blunt-ended nuclei. The cells are uniform with regular nuclei. HE. High magnification. **b** Fragment of collagenous stroma with individual tumour cells. HE. High magnification.

Malignant Tumours

Leiomyosarcoma

Leiomyosarcoma is a common soft tissue sarcoma. All four main clinical variants (retroperitoneal, subcutaneous-cutaneous, deep-seated and originating from large veins) may be referred for FNA. In our experience the subcutaneous-cutaneous or deep subcutaneous tumours are most often needled.

Histopathology

The typical pattern is fascicles of spindle cells with eosinophilic cytoplasm and cigar-shaped, ovoid or rounded nuclei. Nuclear segmentation and paranuclear vacuoles are also features associated with leiomyosarcoma cells. Nuclei in tandem position and nuclear palisading may also occur. The stroma may be focally or extensively myxoid or hyalinized. High-grade malignant leiomyosarcoma often exhibits marked

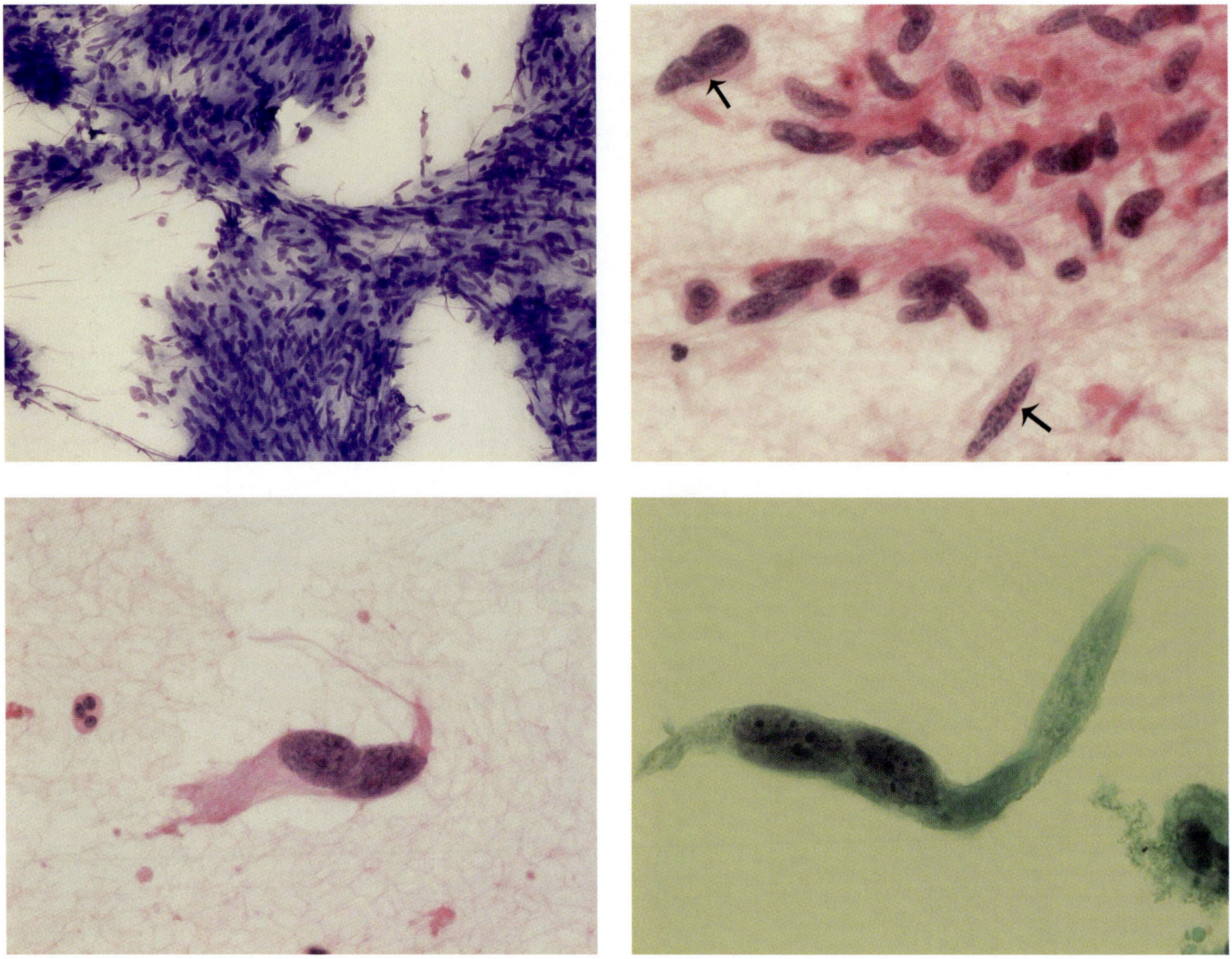

Fig. 41. Leiomyosarcoma, fascicular pattern. **a** Fascicular fragments of cohesive cells. Note the few dispersed large cells in the background. MGG. Low magnification. **b** Moderately pleomorphic elongated, blunt-ended, cigar-shaped or truncated (arrows) nuclei. HE. High magnification. **c** Nuclei in 'tandem position'. HE. High magnification. **d** Nuclei in 'tandem position', ThinPrep preparation. Pap. High magnification.

pleomorphism with the presence of multinucleated tumour giant cells, admixture of osteoclast-like giant cells and necrosis.

In FNA smears three different patterns are present: predominantly fascicular, predominantly pleomorphic and fascicular/pleomorphic. One series of the cytological-histological correlation of leiomyosarcoma has been published [30].

Cytological features of leiomyosarcoma, predominantly fascicular pattern (fig. 41a–d)

- Very variable yield; sarcomas with hyaline degeneration difficult to aspirate
- Fascicular fragments and cellular aggregates of cohesive cells
- Magenta-coloured or blue background matrix in cellular aggregates and fascicles
- Cytoplasmic borders indistinct in aggregates and fascicles
- Moderately pleomorphic elongated nuclei of which many are blunt-ended, cigar-shaped and truncated; nuclei in 'tandem position'
- Often coarse nuclear chromatin, nucleoli may be prominent
- Variable presence of dispersed cells, often with large hyperchromatic, degenerate stripped nuclei

Differential diagnosis

- Deep leiomyoma
- Neurilemoma (especially ancient neurilemoma)
- Desmoid fibromatosis
- MPNST

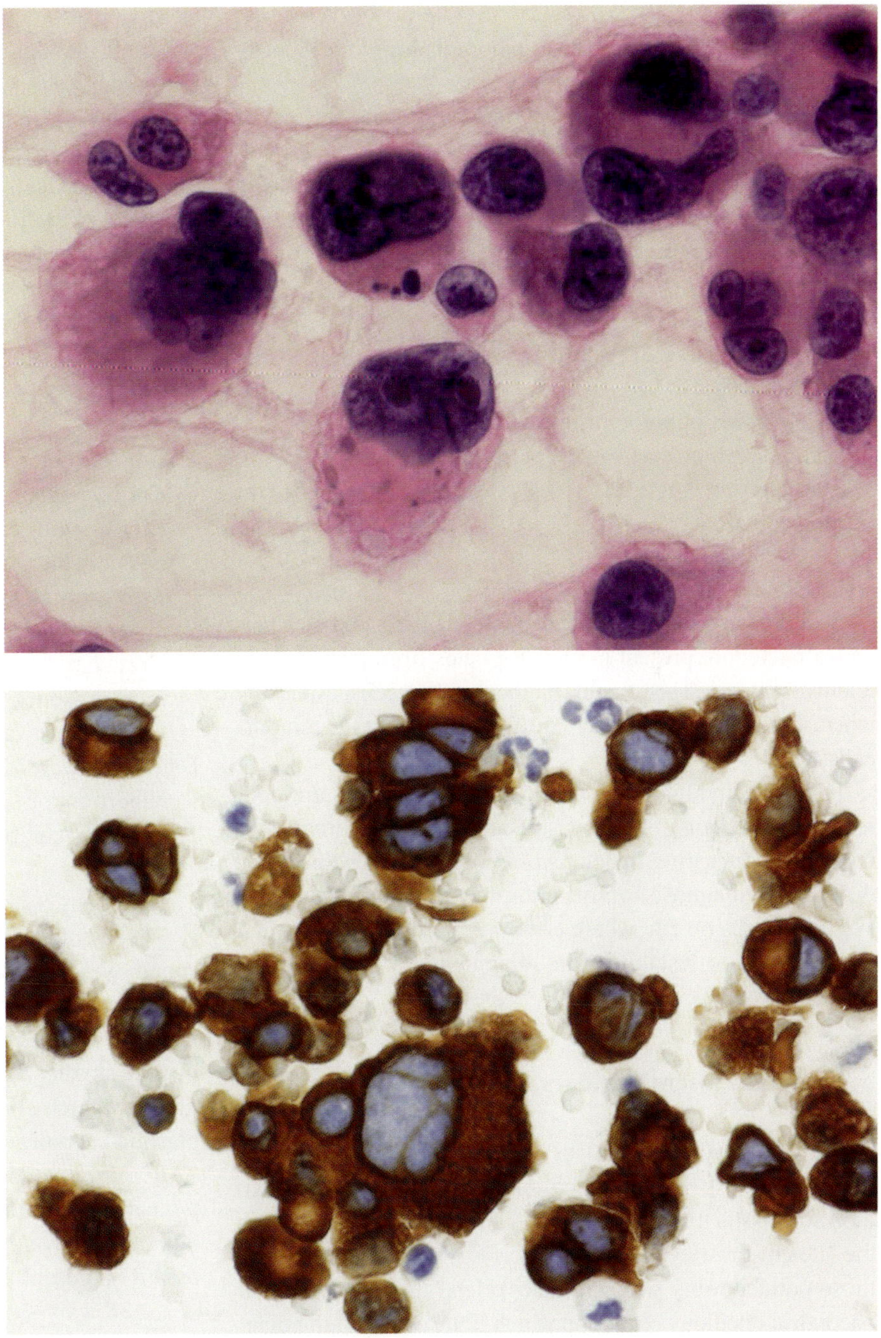

Fig. 42. Leiomyosarcoma, pleomorphic pattern. **a** Marked cellular and nuclear pleomorphism with the presence of multinucleated tumour cells with mainly rounded nuclei. HE. High magnification. **b** Immunocytochemical staining with antidesmin may help to make a specific diagnosis of leiomyosarcoma in a case of pleomorphic sarcoma. Cell block preparation. High magnification.

Comments

The cellular atypia is generally less marked in deep leiomyoma. The presence of mitosis (even a single one) suggests leiomyosarcoma. Neurilemoma is an important pitfall as the spindle cell nuclei in some leiomyosarcomas aspirates are thin, elongated, wavy or have pointed ends. There is a risk of mistakenly diagnosing desmoid fibromatosis if the yield from a leiomyosarcoma is scanty.

IC is helpful in the differential diagnosis. Leiomyosarcomas are negative for S-100 protein and extensive positivity for desmin or caldesmon excludes desmoid. EM is also a valuable adjunct displaying filaments with focal densities, pinocytosis and external laminae.

Cytological features of leiomyosarcoma; pleomorphic pattern (fig. 42a, b)

Dispersed cells and cell clusters; few fascicular fragments

Necrosis
Marked cellular and nuclear pleomorphism; multinucleated tumour cells
Preserved cells often have abundant grey-blue (MGG) or eosinophilic (wet-fixed smear) cytoplasm
Atypical spindle cells; variable amount of tumour cells of 'smooth muscle type'
Variable numbers of rounded cells with atypical rounded nuclei
Epithelioid-like cells
Osteoclast-like giant cells may be present

Differential diagnosis
Other types of pleomorphic sarcoma
Soft tissue metastasis of anaplastic carcinoma
Soft tissue metastasis of sarcomatous malignant melanoma

Comment

Scattered atypical spindle cells with cigar-shaped or blunt-ended nuclei are present in most aspirates from pleomorphic leiomyosarcoma. The rounded epithelioid-like cells, especially when in small clusters, may be misinterpreted as carcinoma cells.

IC is of help although focal positivity for keratin antibodies may be seen in leiomyosarcoma. Focal positivity for myoglobin (negative in leiomyosarcoma) is of help in the differential diagnosis of pleomorphic rhabdomyosarcoma. We have cases on file where electron-microscopic examination helped to establish the diagnosis of pleomorphic leiomyosarcoma.

Skeletal Muscle Tumours

Benign (rhabdomyoma) as well as malignant (rhabdomyosarcoma) skeletal muscle tumours are generally uncommon soft tissue tumours. Only very few cases are recorded in the files of most cytology laboratories with the exception of those collaborating with musculoskeletal tumour centres or paediatric oncology centres in which FNA is part of the diagnostic workup.

Of the various rhabdomyoma entities, adult rhabdomyoma is the most commonly needled one.

Benign Tumours

Adult Rhabdomyoma

Adult rhabdomyoma is most common after the age of 40 and is typically found in the head and neck region. The tongue and the floor of mouth are favoured sites.

Histopathology

Adult rhabdomyomas are composed of large rounded and polygonal cells with abundant eosinophilic granular cytoplasm and small nuclei with prominent nucleoli. The cytoplasm is often vacuolated due to dissolved glycogen. Cross striation is focally present in most tumours and intracytoplasmic crystalline structures are found in many cases. Immunohistochemically the cells stain for desmin, myoglobin, and muscle-specific actin. S-100 protein positivity has been described focally.

Adult rhabdomyoma in FNA smears has been described in individual cases [88, 89].

Cytological features of adult rhabdomyoma (fig. 43a, b)
Large elongated or rounded cells with abundant eosinophilic cytoplasm (wet-fixed smear) and small nuclei with prominent nucleoli
Stripped nuclei common
Granulated cytoplasm, cross striation rare (in spite of the focal presence in tissue sections)
Cytoplasmic vacuoles

Differential diagnosis
Hibernoma
Granular cell tumour

Comment

The cytological features of adult rhabdomyoma correspond well with those seen in tissue sections. Although hibernoma cells in FNA smears are granulated and vacuolated, they are generally smaller than rhabdomyoma cells and display smaller cytoplasmic vacuoles. Cells of granular cell tumour, which also often involves the tongue, have no cytoplasmic vacuoles.

IC is of diagnostic help. Diffuse S-100 protein staining is typical for granular cell tumour, while desmin and myoglobin are negative. If S-100 protein is expressed in rhabdomyoma it is present focally.

Malignant Tumours

Rhabdomyosarcoma

During the last decade various suggestions have been made as regards the classification of rhabdomyosarcoma. At present four classifications are in use: the modified conventional classification, the International Society for Paediatric Oncology Classification (SIOP), the National Cancer Institute Classification (NCI) and the International Classification of Rhabdomyosarcoma (ICR) [90, 91]. Common to all are

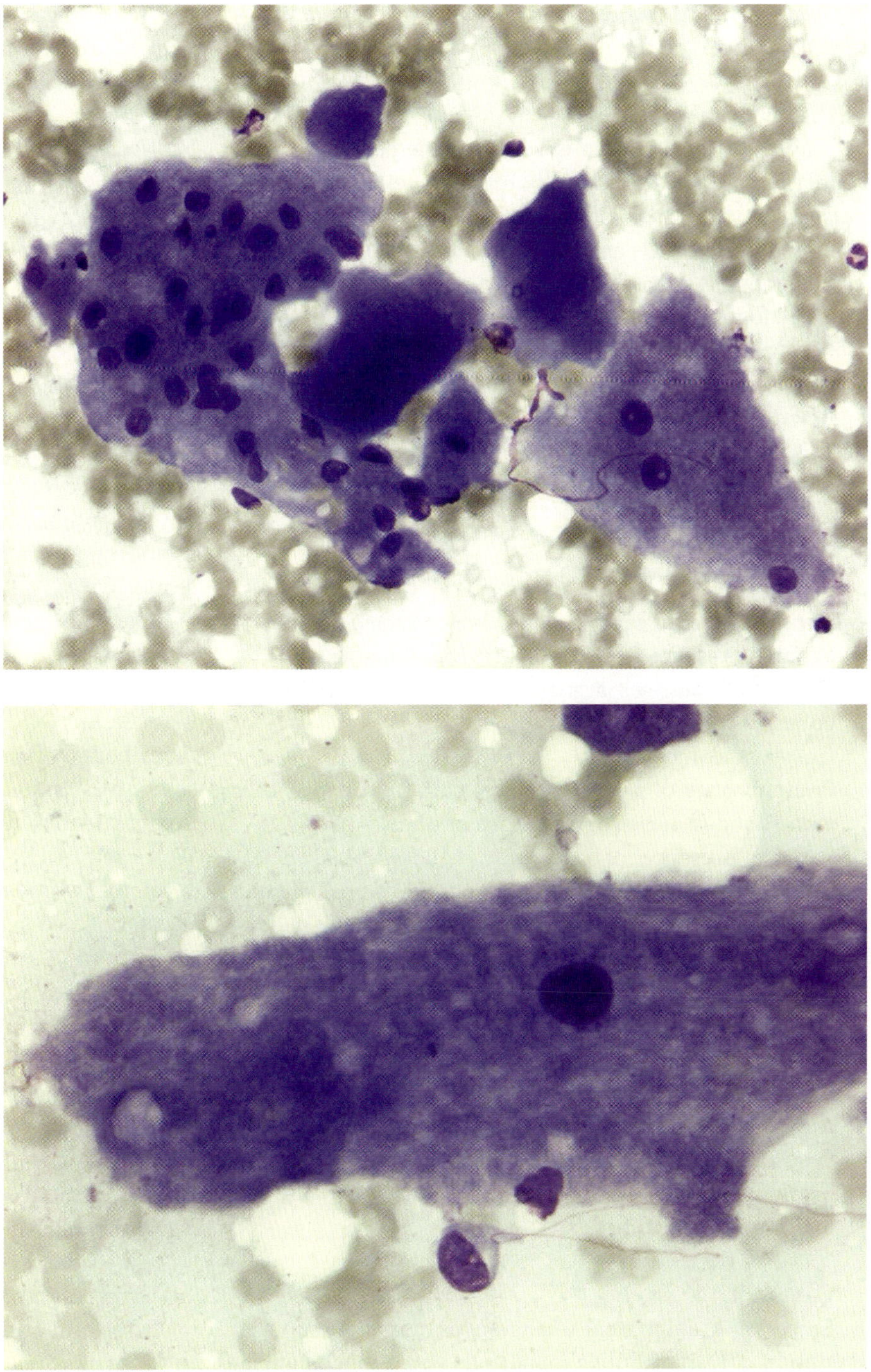

a

b

Fig. 43. Adult rhabdomyoma. **a** Large, cytoplasm-rich rounded and polygonal cells with deep-blue cytoplasm and multiple small nuclei. MGG. High magnification. **b** A large elongated rhabdomyoma cell with granulated cytoplasm. MGG. High magnification.

the three main 'classic' subtypes: embryonal, alveolar and pleomorphic.

The NCI and ICR classifications stress that embryonal rhabdomyosarcoma (all variants) belong to a prognostically favourable group while the alveolar type, including all rhabdomyosarcomas showing an alveolar pattern focally, are considered prognostically unfavourable. Pure pleomorphic rhabdomyosarcoma is an aggressive sarcoma in adults.

Embryonal Rhabdomyosarcoma

Close to 50% of all rhabdomyosarcoma are embryonal, most common in children below the age of 10. The most common sites are the head and neck region, genitourinary tract and pelvis and retroperitoneum.

Histopathology

The histological pattern is very variable as regards both cellularity, presence of myxoid areas and cellular pleomorphism. The cellular composition is a blend of rounded or spindly primitive cells and rhabdomyoblast-like cells, which may be tadpole-shaped, strap-shaped, triangular or rounded. The predominantly paratesticular spindle cell variant of embryonal rhabdomyosarcoma is principally composed of eosinophilic spindle cells.

Practically all embryonal rhabdomyosarcomas stain for desmin, muscle-specific actin, MyoD1 and myogenin. The cytological appearance of embryonal rhabdomyosarcoma has been reported [40, 44].

Cytological features of embryonal rhabdomyosarcoma (fig. 44a–c)

Variable presence of myxoid background matrix
Dispersed cells, cell aggregates and clusters of loosely cohesive cells
Cellular pleomorphism
Predominance of primitive spindle cells or rounded cells with rounded nuclei, or a mixture of both
Variable presence of cells with rhabdomyoblastic features; tadpole-like, strap-shaped, ribbon-like or elongated
Eosinophilic (wet-fixed smear) or grey-blue (MGG) cytoplasm in rhabdomyoblast-like cells
Variable tumour cell chromatin structure; nucleoli may be prominent

Differential diagnosis

Desmoid fibromatosis
Alveolar rhabdomyosarcoma
Synovial sarcoma (monophasic fibrous type)
Leiomyosarcoma
Infantile fibrosarcoma

Comment

Smears of embryonal rhabdomyosarcoma composed predominantly of primitive round cells with rounded nuclei may resemble those of alveolar rhabdomyosarcoma. The cells are, however, larger than those of the alveolar type and anisocytosis and anisokaryosis are more marked. Smears of the spindle cell variant of embryonal rhabdomyosarcoma may consist almost exclusively of atypical spindle cells and typical rhabdomyoblasts may be difficult to find.

One diagnostic pifall is leiomyosarcoma, although this tumour is rare in children. A positive desmin stain excludes non-myogenic spindle cell sarcoma and a positive staining with MyoD1 or myogenin confirms skeletal muscle origin. EM is also a valuable diagnostic asset.

Alveolar Rhabdomyosarcoma

About one third of all rhabdomyosarcomas belong to the alveolar subtype. Alveolar rhabdomyosarcoma is most common between 10 and 25 years of age. The limbs are the favoured site, but the trunk and head and neck region are also common sites.

Histopathology

The dominant neoplastic cells are small- to medium-sized, rounded, ovoid or pear-shaped with round or oval nucleus and scanty cytoplasm. Nuclei are hyperchromatic, occasionally with prominent nucleoli. Multinucleated giant cells with peripherally located nuclei are a common finding in tissue sections.

Like embryonal rhabdomyosarcoma, the alveolar variant is positive for desmin in practically all cases. The majority stain for myogenin and MyoD1. Aberrant expression of cytokeratin, NSE, S-100 protein and CD99 has been described. A specific chromosomal aberration [t(2;13)(q35;q14)] is found in almost all cases of alveolar rhabdomyosarcoma, resulting in a fusion transcript between the PAX3 and FKHR genes.

In many publications alveolar rhabdomyosarcoma has been evaluated cytologically [39–43].

Cytological features of alveolar rhabdomyosarcoma (fig. 45a–g)

Often highly cellular smears
Dispersed cells and clusters of loosely cohesive cells
Many stripped nuclei, blue-grey background of smeared cytoplasm
Preserved cells small- to medium-sized, rounded, ovoid or pear-shaped with scanty cytoplasm; uniform cellular pattern
Coarse chromatin and often prominent nucleoli
Cytoplasmic vacuolation
Mitotic figures
Rhabdomyoblastic differentiation in variable proportion of tumour cells; eccentric nuclei, eosinophilic (wet-fixed smear) or grey-blue (MGG) cytoplasm
Occasionally multinucleated tumour cells

Differential diagnosis

Ewing family of tumours
Neuroblastoma
Poorly differentiated synovial sarcoma
Small-cell malignant melanoma

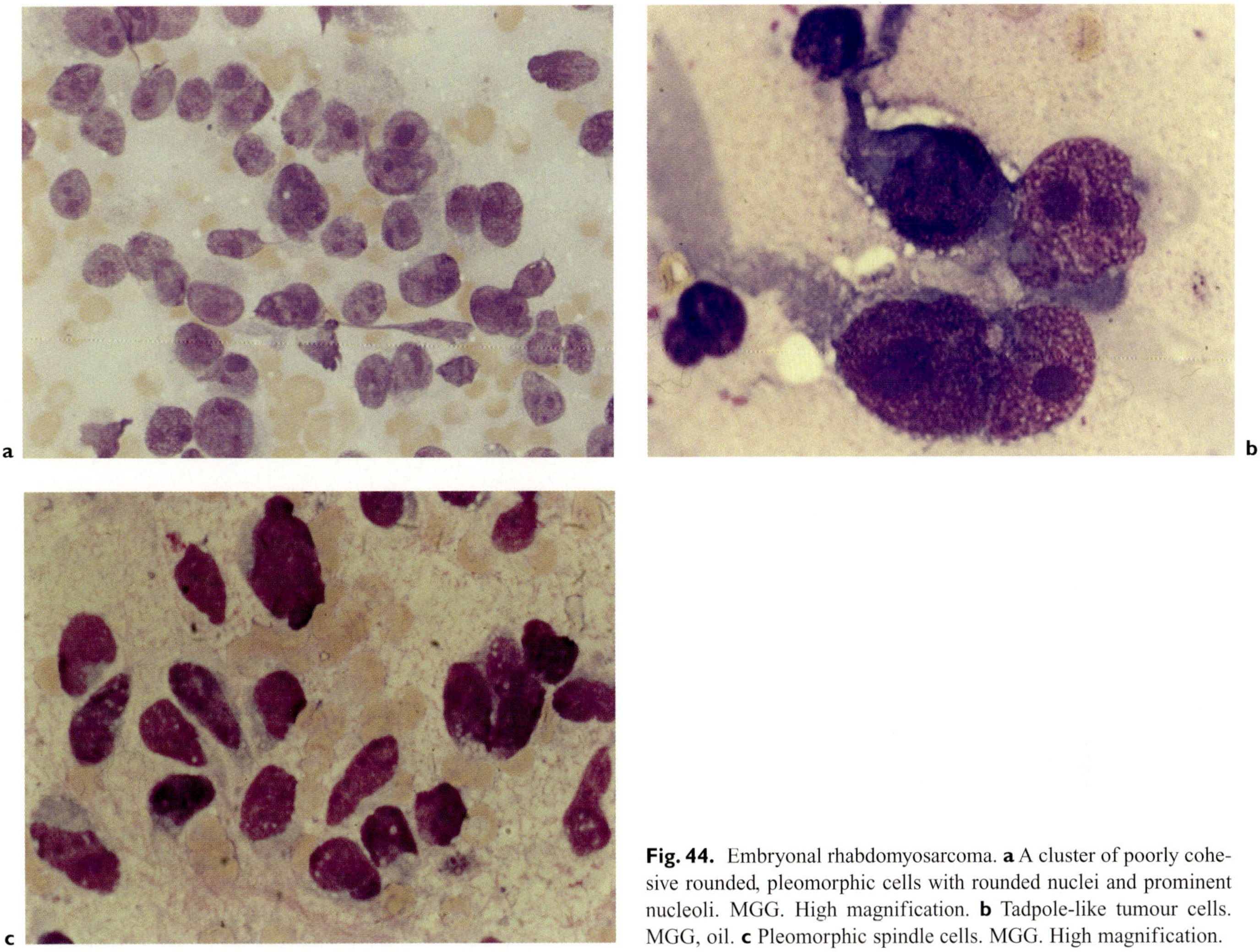

Fig. 44. Embryonal rhabdomyosarcoma. **a** A cluster of poorly cohesive rounded, pleomorphic cells with rounded nuclei and prominent nucleoli. MGG. High magnification. **b** Tadpole-like tumour cells. MGG, oil. **c** Pleomorphic spindle cells. MGG. High magnification.

Precursor lymphoma
Granulocytic sarcoma

Comment

Alveolar rhabdomyosarcoma is a true small round cell malignancy and when definitive treatment is based on FNA the cytological diagnosis should be supplemented with special diagnostic methods. Our experience is similar to others in that IC as well as EM are valuable diagnostic adjuncts. Cytogenetic and molecular genetic analyses are promising diagnostic tools.

As pure alveolar rhabdomyosarcomas and all rhabdomyosarcomas with a focal alveolar pattern are considered therapeutically unfavourable neoplasms, it is clinically important to correctly distinguish between alveolar and embryonal rhabdomyosarcoma in FNA smears. There are different opinions in regard to this subclassification. Our experience corresponds with that of Atahan et al. [40] that it is possible in most cases to subtype rhabdomyosarcoma in embryonal and alveolar variants [92].

Pleomorphic Rhabdomyosarcoma

Pleomorphic rhabdomyosarcoma is the least common of the rhabdomyosarcomas. It is a sarcoma usually found in adults, most often in those older than 50 years. The majority of cases arise in the limbs.

Histopathology

Pleomorphic rhabdomyosarcoma is a high-grade malignant sarcoma exhibiting abundant marked cellular and nuclear atypia cells. It is composed of atypical spindle cells and large, often bizarre tumour eosinophilic cytoplasm. Multinucleated tumour cells are also part of the cellular pattern. Pleomorphic rhabdomyosarcoma is a rare sarcoma and only individual cases are represented in our files.

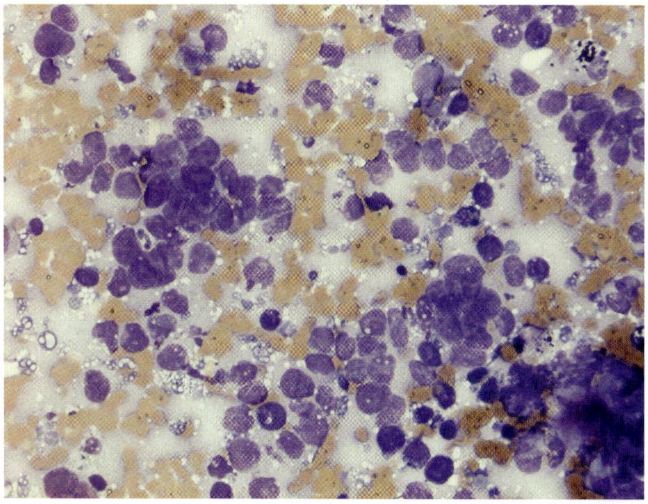

45a

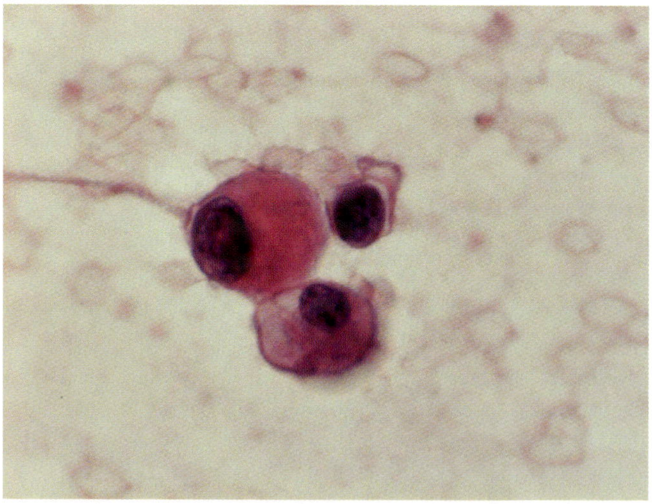

45b

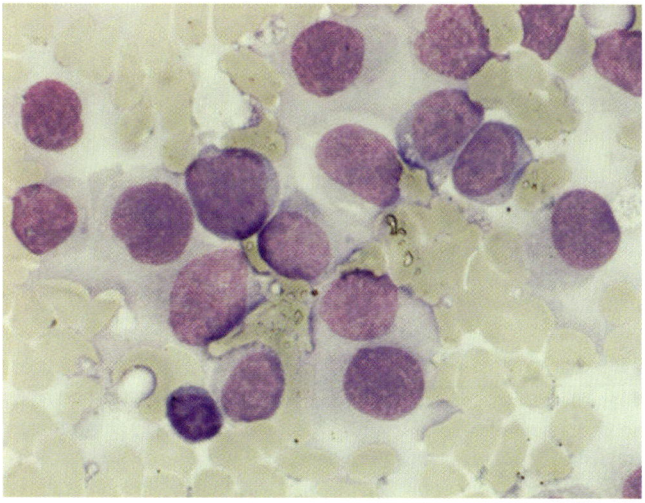

45c

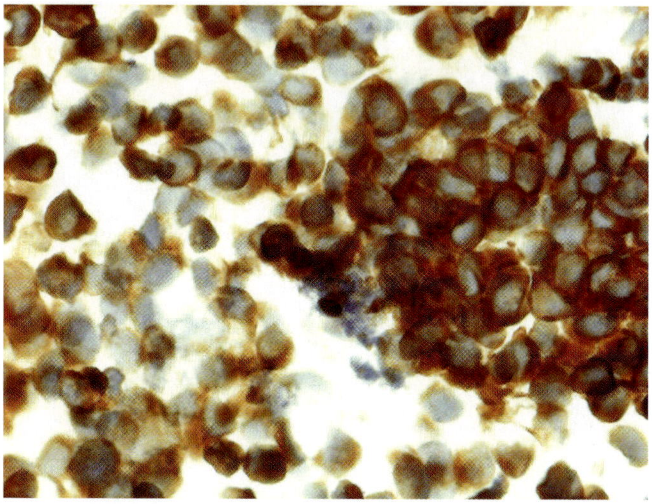

45d

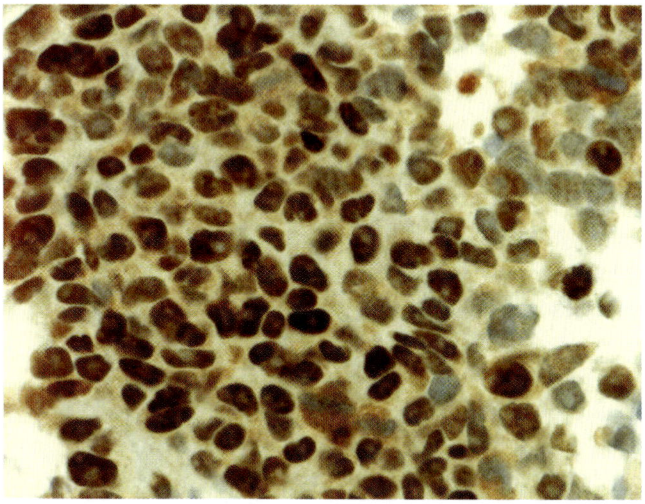

45e

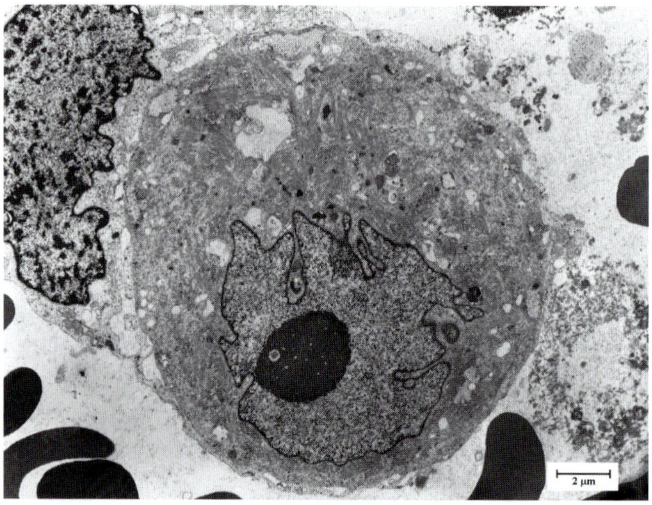

45f

45g 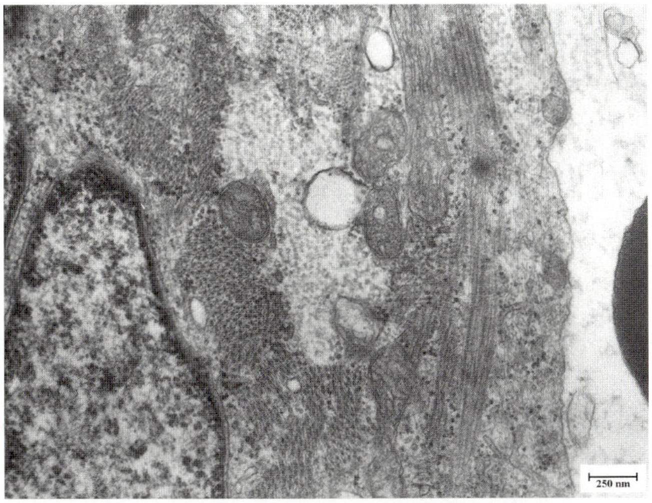

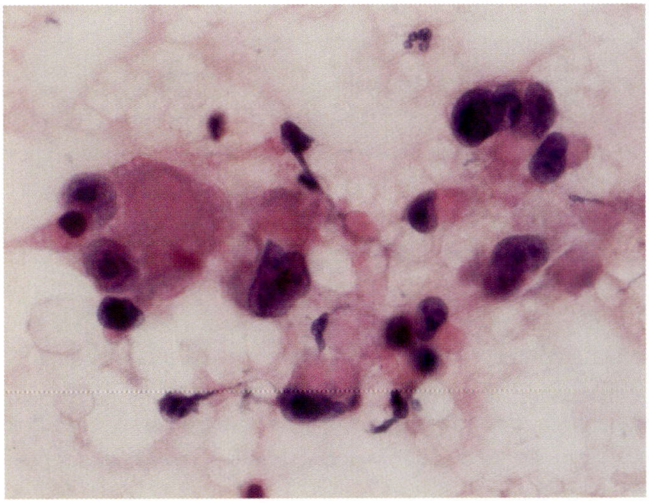 46a

46b 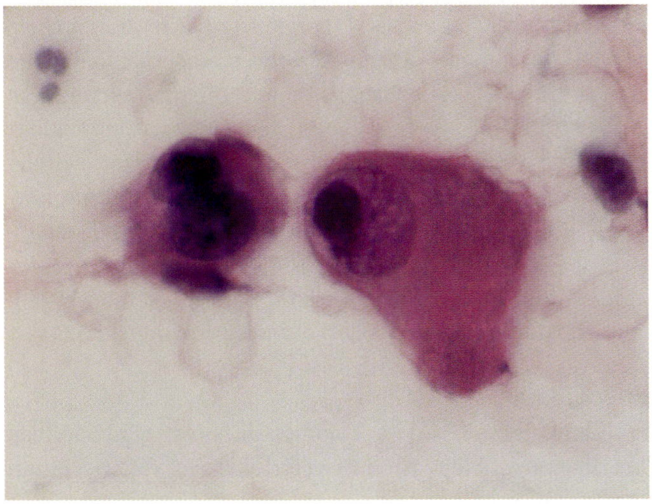

Fig. 45. Alveolar rhabdomyosarcoma. **a** A cellular smear of dispersed cells and cell clusters in a blue-grey background of dispersed cytoplasm. MGG. Low magnification. **b** Typical rhabdomyoblasts. HE. High magnification. **c** MGG. High magnification. **d**, **e** Immunocytochemistry. Strong desmin positivity (**d**) and strong MyoD1 nuclear positivity (**e**) in a cell block preparation. **f** EM examination. Rhabdomyoblast at low magnification. **g** The typical filaments with Z-bands are evident at high magnification.

Fig. 46. Pleomorphic rhabdomyosarcoma. **a**, **b** Large pleomorphic, cytoplasm-rich cells with features of highly atypical rhabdomyoblasts. HE. High magnification.

Cytological features of pleomorphic rhabdomyosarcoma (fig. 46a, b)

Dispersed cells and cell clusters

Marked cellular and nuclear pleomorphism

Atypical spindle cells, large atypical rhabdomyoblast-like cells with abundant eosinophilic cytoplasm (HE), multinucleated tumour cells

Differential diagnosis

Other types of pleomorphic sarcoma

Comment

Pleomorphic rhabdomyosarcoma and pleomorphic leiomyosarcoma may exhibit quite a similar cytomorphology in smears. As desmin is positive in both tumours, specific skeletal muscle markers such as monoclonal myoglobin, MyoD1 and/or myogenin should be included in the antibody panel. The large atypical rhabdomyoblast-like cells are often, at least focally, myoglobin positive.

Tumours of Peripheral Nerves

Among the various benign tumours and lesions of peripheral nerves, neurilemoma (schwannoma) is the most common in FNA-files. Neurofibromas are occasionally biopsied, especially in patients with von Recklinghausen's disease and growing tumours which are referred with a question of malignant transformation. There are individual reports of FNA of the rare perineurioma, while case reports and a few series of granular cell tumour have been published. MPNST are infrequently subjected to FNA, and many of those needled are associated with von Recklinghausen's disease.

Benign Tumours

Neurilemoma (Schwannoma)

Neurilemomas occur in all age groups but are most frequent in persons between 20 and 50 years of age. They occur in any part of the body but the most common sites are the limbs, the head and neck region, retroperitoneum and posterior mediastinum.

Among the five major benign tumours, lipoma, neurilemoma, intramuscular myxoma, desmoid fibromatosis and haemangioma, neurilemoma is the second most frequently aspirated after lipoma according to our files. The cytomorphology as reported [20–22] is predominantly based on the evaluation of histological Antoni A areas in surgical specimens.

Cytological features of neurilemoma, Antoni A component (fig. 47a–f)

Tumour fragments of different sizes with irregular borders; 'pieces of a jig saw puzzle'
Few dispersed cells
Variable cellularity in fragments
The tumour cells in fragments have indistinct cytoplasm, nuclei are embedded in a fibrillary background
Nuclear palisading variable
Typical nuclei are long and slender, comma- or boomerang-shaped with pointed ends
Small rounded lymphocyte-like nuclei may be part of the cell population
Moderate nuclear pleomorphism; bland chromatin structure
Occasionally Verocay-like bodies

Cytological features of neurilemoma, Antoni B component

Variable presence of myxoid background and cystic degeneration
Mainly dispersed cells, few small tissue fragments
Inflammatory cells, histiocytes
Variable proportions of Antoni A and Antoni B features are present in most samples of neurilemoma

Differential diagnosis

Spindle cell lipoma
Solitary fibrous tumour
Low-grade malignant MPNST
Leiomyosarcoma
Myxoid soft tissue tumours (cases with abundant myxoid background matrix)

Comment

The needling of most neurilemomas triggers a sharp pain, often radiating along the nerve. This is a valuable diagnostic sign but the same type of pain may be encountered when needling other types of soft tissue tumour situated close to a nerve.

The most important pitfall is to misinterpret neurilemoma aspirates as malignant, as MPNST or leiomyosarcoma. This is above all the case with ancient neurilemoma [93, 94], which exhibits marked anisokaryosis and hyperchromatic, large nuclei. However, the large nuclei are degenerate with typical large nuclear vacuoles, 'kern-loch', and it is usually possible to find typical Antoni A fragments in the smears (fig. 48a–c). IC is of diagnostic help. S-100 protein positivity indicates a peripheral nerve sheath tumour while positive staining for desmin and/or smooth muscle actin indicates a smooth muscle tumour. S-100 protein positivity is of no help in the differential diagnosis between neurilemoma and low-grade MPNST. Usually the tumour fragments in MPNST are homogenously cellular, the nuclear chromatin is coarser and more hyperchromatic. The variant cellular schwannoma is especially difficult to distinguish from low-grade MPNST in smears [95]. However, cellular schwannomas are always positive for S-100 protein in almost every cell, while MPNST often stain focally or not at all. Individual mitotic figures do not indicate malignancy.

Neurofibroma

Neurofibroma is less common in FNA material than neurilemoma. Most patients referred have von Recklinghausen's disease.

Histopathology

The stroma in neurofibroma is usually fibromyxoid but may be collagenous or hyalinized. The lesional cells are spindle-shaped with bent, wavy or comma-shaped slender nuclei. Degenerate areas may show similar nuclear characteristics as in ancient neurilemoma.

Neurofibroma is infrequently described in the cytological literature [22].

Cytological features of neurofibroma (fig. 49a, b)

Variable yield (due to the content of collagen)
Variable amount of myxoid background substance
Stripped nuclei
Dispersed cells and loose clusters
Spindle cells with elongated nuclei, mixture of cells with Schwann cell characteristics (wavy, irregular nuclei, nuclei with pointed ends) and fibroblast-like cells
Bland chromatin structure

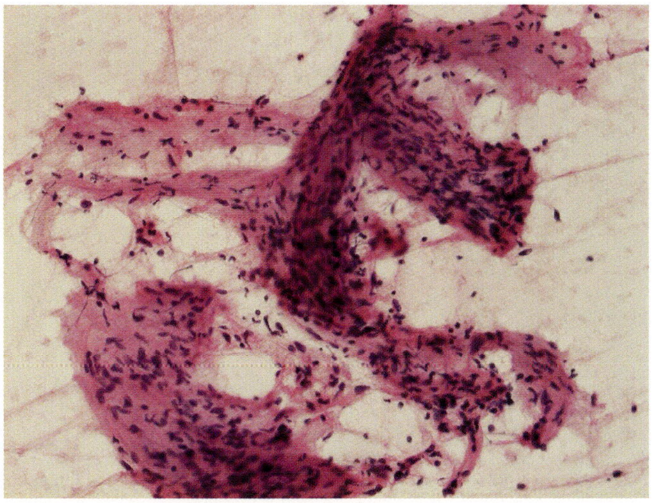
47a

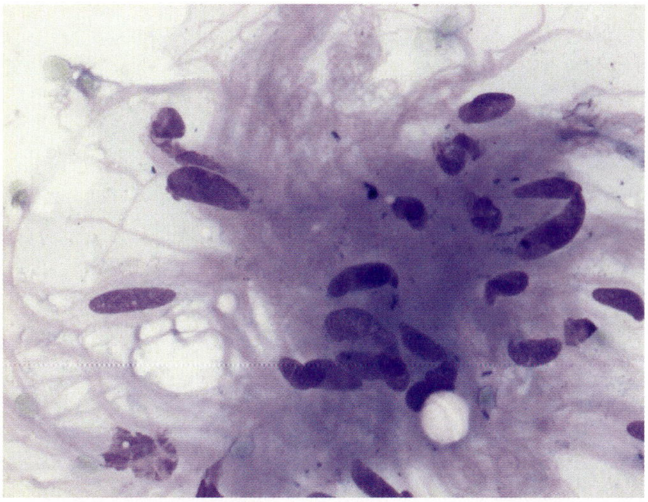
47b

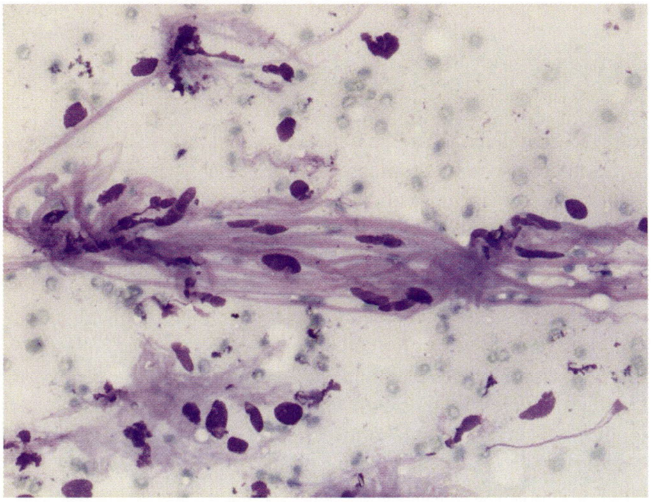
47c

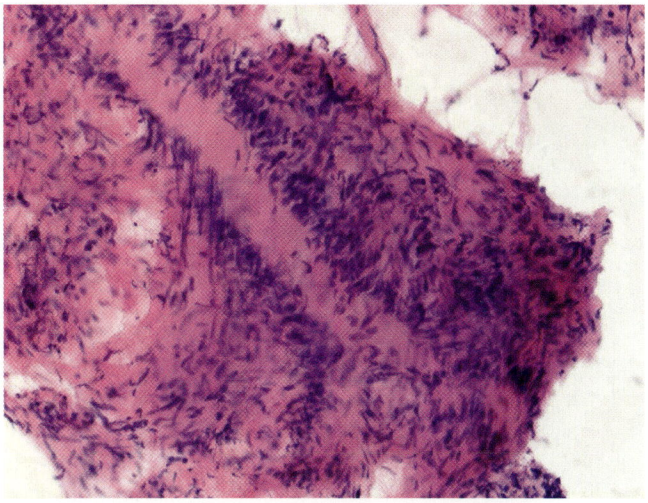
47d

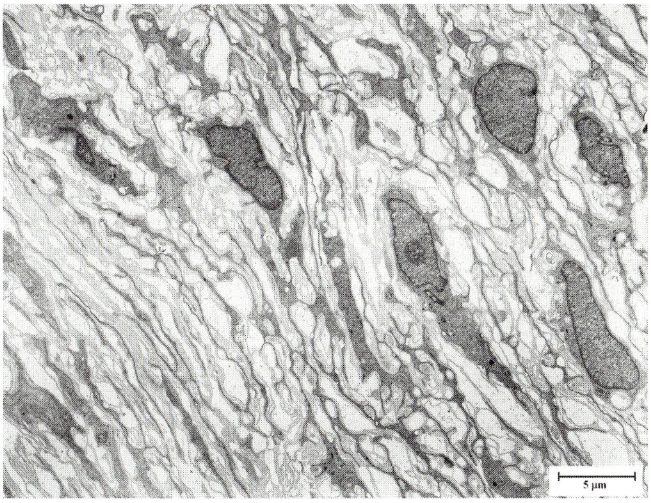

47e

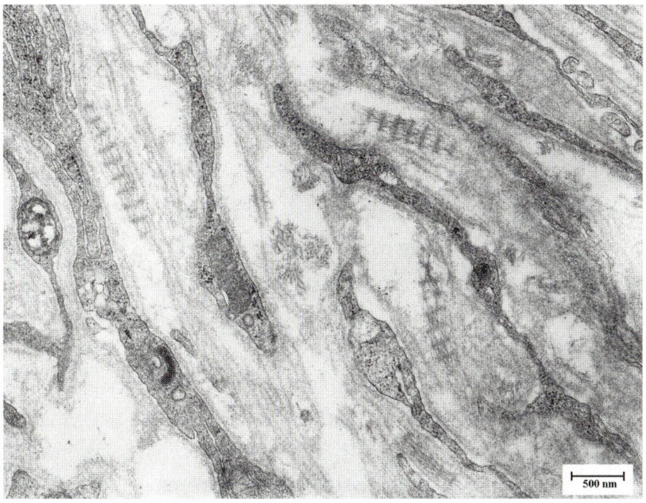

47f

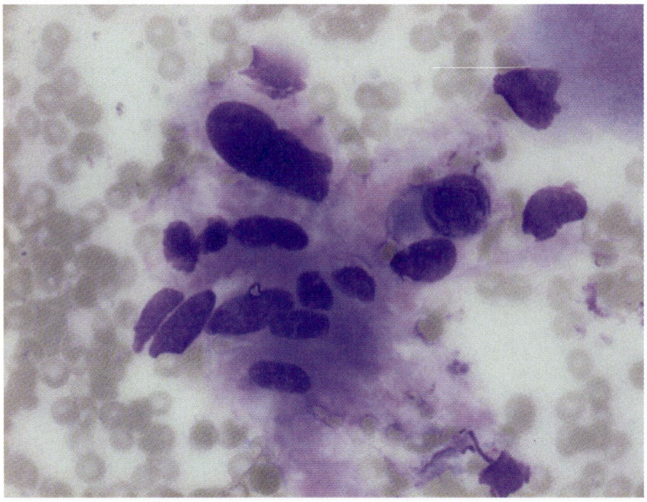

48a

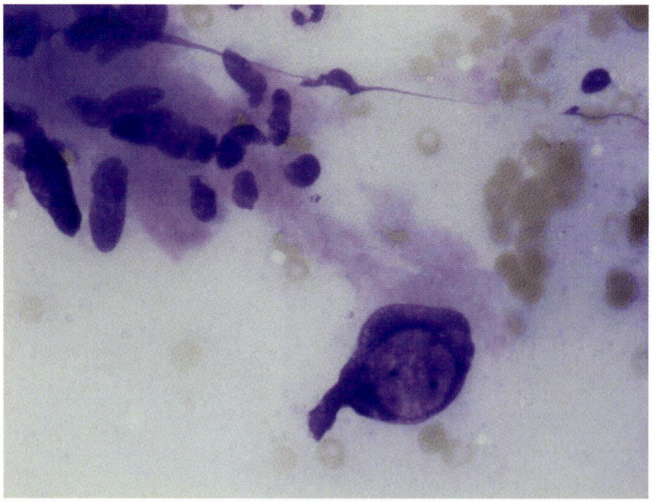

48b

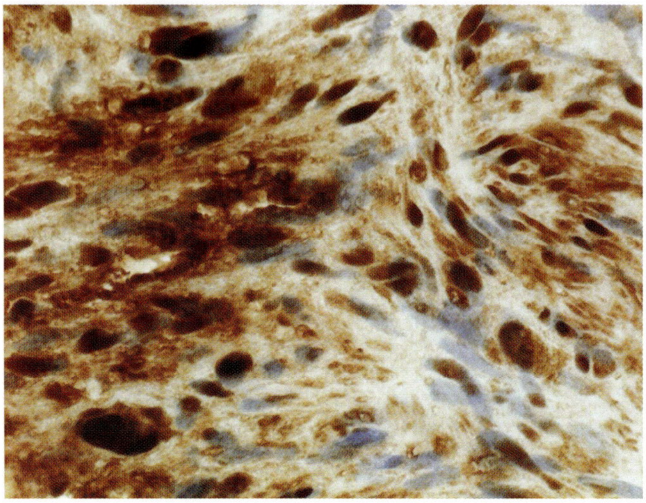

48c

Fig. 47. Neurilemoma. **a** The typical appearance of neurilemoma in a smear under low power: variably cellular, variably sized tumour fragments. HE. Low magnification. **b**, **c** The tumour cells have indistinct cytoplasm and the nuclei are embedded in a fibrillary background. MGG. High magnification. **d** A Verocay-like body. HE. Low magnification. **e** EM preparation of an FNA biopsy from a neurilemoma in low magnification. Cells with spindly nuclei connected by interdigitating cell processes. **f** Between the cells bundles of long spaced collagen.

Fig. 48. Ancient neurilemoma. **a** Marked anisokaryosis, hyperchromatic nuclei. MGG. High magnification. **b** One of the nuclei in this cluster shows a 'kern-loch'. MGG. High magnification. **c** Positive S-100 protein staining in an ancient neurilemoma. Cell block preparation.

Differential diagnosis

Neurilemoma with a predominant Antoni B component
Intramuscular myxoma
Solitary fibrous tumour
Spindle cell lipoma
Low-grade myxofibrosarcoma
Low-grade MPNST

Comment

Neurofibroma with abundant myxoid matrix may be falsely diagnosed as a number of other myxoid neoplasms. Neurofibroma with atypical cells may be misinterpreted as low-grade malignant MPNST. Neurofibroma is a difficult cytological diagnosis. It is most commonly diagnosed as 'benign myxoid spindle cell tumour'. A variable amount of the spindle cells stains for S-100 protein.

Granular Cell Tumour

Granular cell tumours occur in any age group, but are most common in middle-aged people. They are rare in children. They are more often subcutaneous than deeply localized. The tongue is a fairly common site and granular cell tumours in the breast are often needled in the diagnostic workup of breast lesions. A comprehensive study of the cytological features of benign and malignant granular cell tumour has been published [23].

Histopathology

Granular tumour cells are rounded, polygonal or spindly with abundant eosinophilic, granular cytoplasm. The nuclei vary between small and dark or large and vesicular. A moderate degree of nuclear atypia is not uncommon.

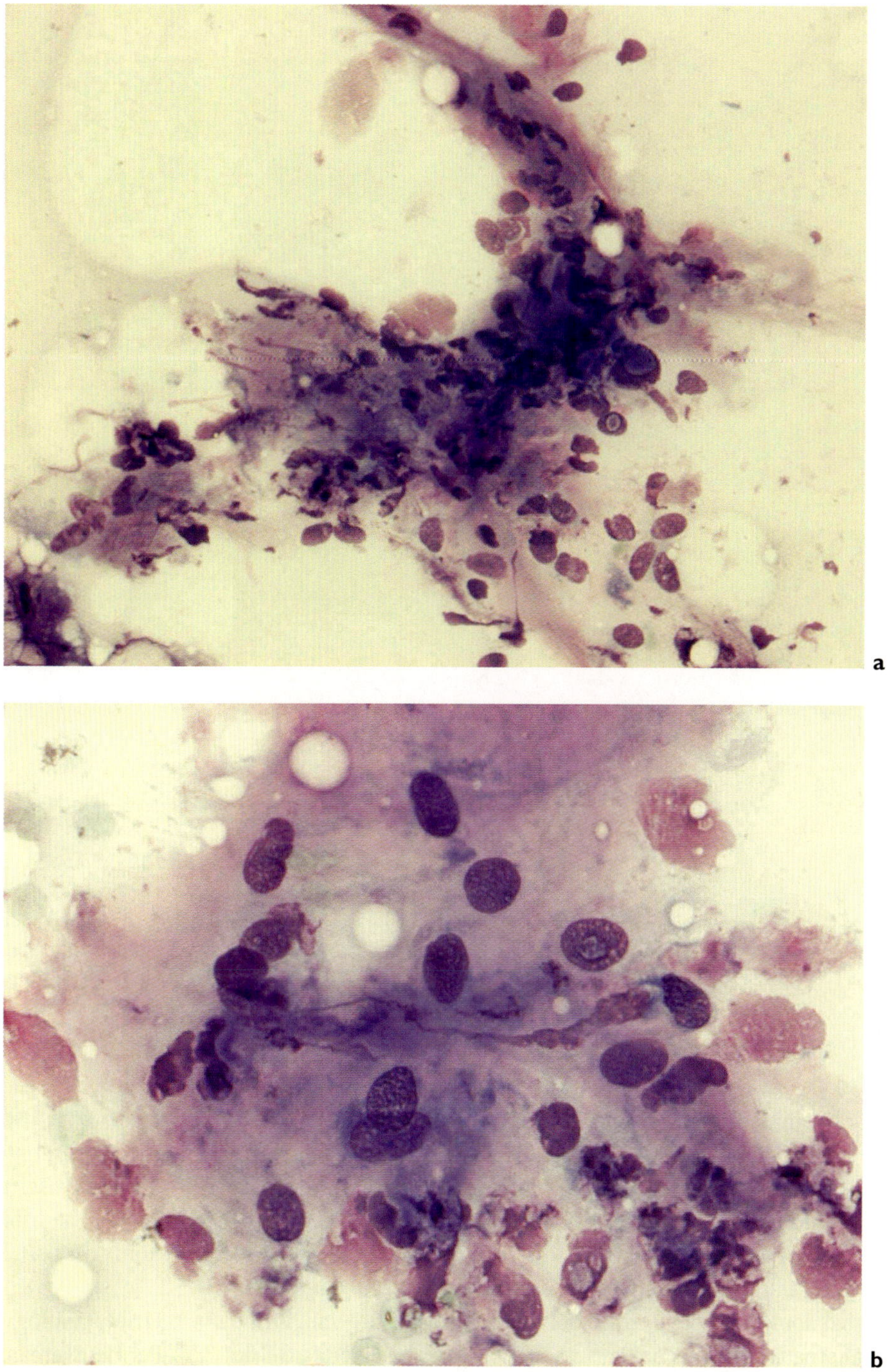

Fig. 49. Neurofibroma. **a** Myxoid background in tumour fragment composed of rounded and spindle-shaped cells. MGG. Low magnification. **b** Often, the tumour cell population is dominated by fibroblast-like cells. MGG. Medium magnification.

Cytological features of granular cell tumour (fig. 50a–c)

Individual cells and cells in cohesive clusters

Stripped nuclei and cytoplasmic granular background commonly seen

Preserved cells are rounded, polygonal or spindly with abundant granular cytoplasm

Preserved cells have indistinct cytoplasmic borders

Nuclei are mainly small, rounded, with finely granular chromatin and small nucleoli

A number of cells with larger nuclei with coarse chromatin and large nucleoli is present in almost every case

Differential diagnosis

Hibernoma

Adult rhabdomyoma

Alveolar soft part sarcoma

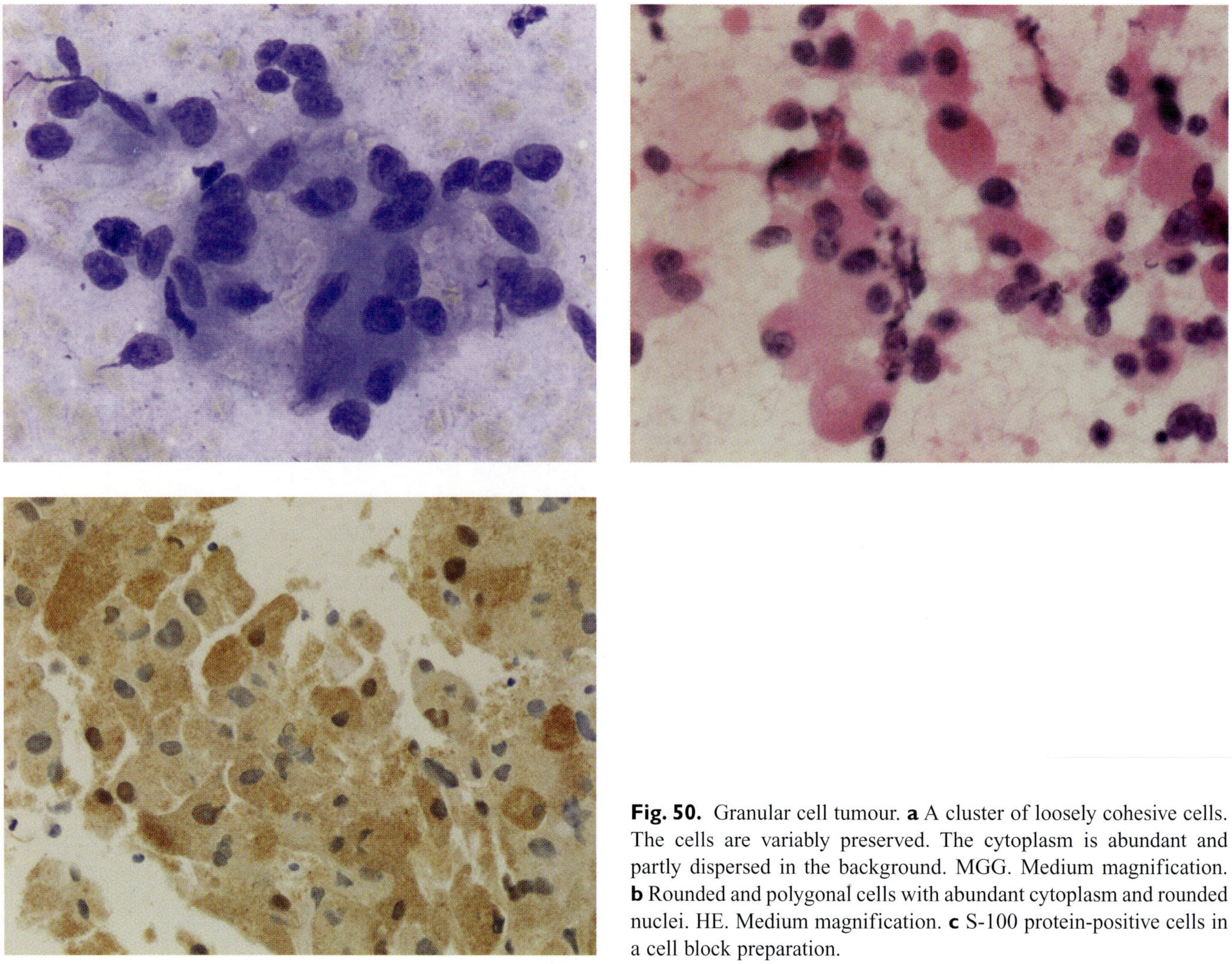

Fig. 50. Granular cell tumour. **a** A cluster of loosely cohesive cells. The cells are variably preserved. The cytoplasm is abundant and partly dispersed in the background. MGG. Medium magnification. **b** Rounded and polygonal cells with abundant cytoplasm and rounded nuclei. HE. Medium magnification. **c** S-100 protein-positive cells in a cell block preparation.

Comment

The granulated hibernoma cells resemble granular tumour cells but in hibernoma smears there is most often a mixed population of ordinary fat cells and hibernoma cells, of which many are vacuolated.

IC and EM of aspirated material give diagnostic clues when rhabdomyoma or alveolar soft part sarcoma are diagnostic alternatives. The granular tumour cells are positive for S-100 protein and NSE and have characteristic ultrastructural features, i.e. innumerable lysosomes filled with osmiophilic material.

Perineurioma

Perineurioma is a rare soft tissue tumour, the cells of which resemble perineurial cells of normal perineurium. Cytopathologists might come across the soft tissue (extraneural) perineurioma. The few cases reported have occurred in adults, most commonly in the superficial soft tissues.

Due to its myxoid matrix perineurioma is one of the numerous soft tissue tumour entities exhibiting an abundance of myxoid background substance in FNA material and represents a differential diagnostic alternative among the myxoid soft tissue tumours.

Histopathology

Perineurioma is composed of slender spindle cells arranged in fascicles or a storiform pattern. The cellularity is variable as is the type of stroma. The stroma might be prominently myxoid or more or less collagenized. The tumour cells have long, thin cytoplasmic processes.

Immunohistochemically the perineurioma cells are EMA-positive like normal perineurial cells. They are S-100 protein negative. At electron-microscopic examination slender elongated cells with thin cytoplasmic processes containing pinocytotic vesicles are seen. The cells are invested with basal laminae.

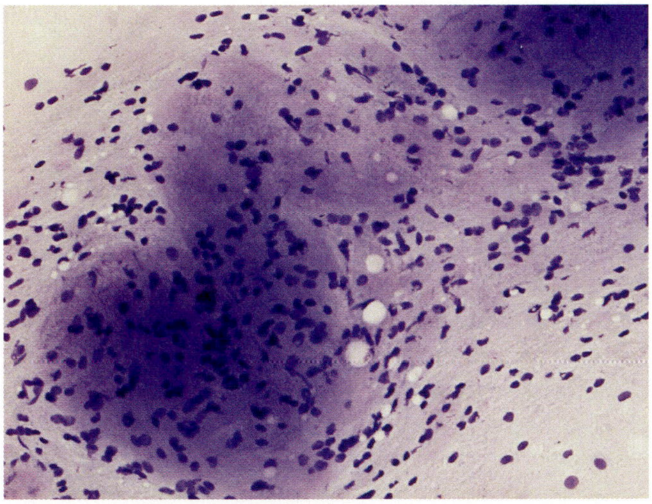
a

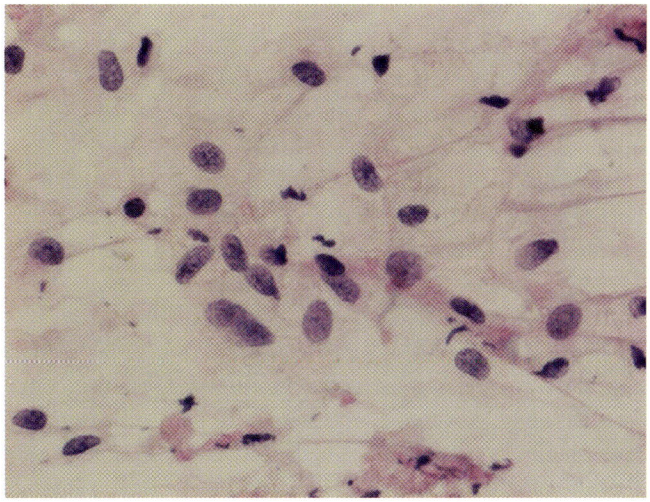
b

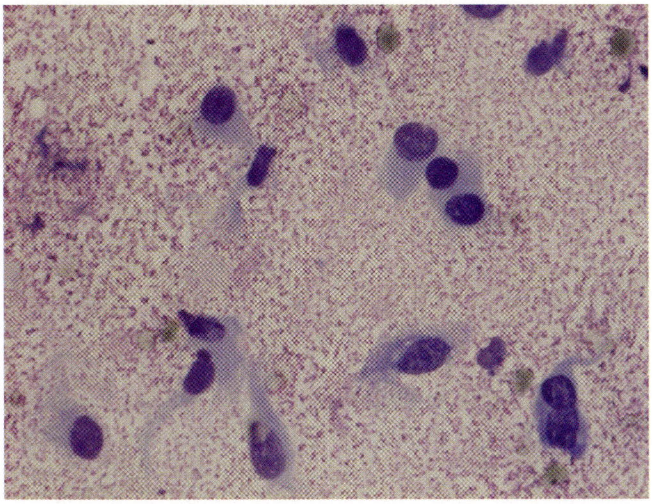
c

Fig. 51. Perineurioma. **a** Dispersed and clustered tumour cells in a myxoid background matrix. Perineurioma shares this appearance in smears at low magnification with several other 'myxoid' soft tissue tumours. MGG. Low magnification. **b** The elongated intact tumour cells have long cytoplasmic processes and bland nuclei. HE. Medium magnification. **c** A group of perineurioma cells. The myxoid matrix is more obvious in MGG-stained smears. MGG. Medium magnification.

The cytological features of perineurioma have been described in a single case [96]; the microscopic features listed below are collected from that case report and our individual cases.

Cytological features of perineurioma (fig. 51a–c)
- Abundant myxoid background matrix
- Variable cellularity
- Elongated cells with ovoid, fusiform or rounded nuclei
- Many stripped nuclei
- Intact cells have long, thin bipolar cytoplasmic processes
- Moderate anisokaryosis
- Uniform chromatin structure
- Scattered vessel fragments in the background matrix

Differential diagnosis
- Neurilemoma with predominant Antoni B areas with abundant myxoid background matrix
- Neurofibroma
- Intramuscular myxoma
- Low-grade myxofibrosarcoma
- Fibromyxoid low-grade sarcoma

Comment

Aspirates from perineurioma are most commonly diagnosed as 'benign myxoid soft tissue tumours' although the cellularity and anisokaryosis might be misinterpreted as indicating a low-grade myxoid sarcoma. A specific diagnosis of perineurioma is most probably not possible without the help of IC and/or EM.

Malignant Tumours

Malignant Peripheral Nerve Sheath Tumour

MPNST include those malignant tumours which arise from the different cells of the nerve sheath (Schwann cells, perineural cells, fibroblasts). It is estimated that MPNST constitute 5–10% of the soft tissue sarcomas. The majority originate from neurofibroma or arise in peripheral nerves. Patients are usually adults, but MPNST may occur in children and adolescents. Patients with neurofibromatosis have an increased risk of developing MPNST.

MPNST more often arise from medium-sized and large nerves than from smaller nerves. The thigh, buttock, upper arm, brachial plexus and paraspinal nerves are the predominant sites.

Histopathology

The histological features of MPNST are very variable. Most appear as spindle cell sarcomas, more or less fibrosarcoma-like. Fascicles, a whorled arrangement of cells or a storiform pattern, are common patterns under low power. Cellular fascicles alternating with hypocellular areas are a common finding. The tumour cell is elongated and has a fusiform nucleus with tapered or rounded ends. Wavy, buckled or comma-shaped nuclei are typical features. Pleomorphic and multinucleated tumour cells are found in a number of cases. Heterotopic elements are present in 10–15% of tumours, most commonly islands of mature bone and cartilage. Skeletal muscle and glandular elements are rare.

Immunohistochemically, S-100 protein positivity is present in between 30 and 70% of tumours, the staining is often focal and there may be a small number of positive cells. CD57 is reported to stain a large number of MPNSTs but unfortunately other spindle cell sarcomas such as synovial sarcoma and leiomyosarcoma may also be positive.

MPNSTs are characterized by many of the same ultrastructural features as are seen in benign nerve sheath tumours. Branching cytoplasmic processes containing microtubuli and filaments are present as well as the coating of cells with basal lamina. Long-spacing collagen is yet another feature.

The literature on FNA cytology of MPNST is rather extensive but mainly as reports of individual cases. Two relatively large series of the cytomorphology of MPNST have been published [33, 34].

Cytological features of MPNST (fig. 52a–d)

- Dispersed cells and cell clusters or fascicles in variable proportions most common pattern
- A fibrillary background may be seen in clusters and fascicles
- Spindle-shaped cells with elongated, wavy or comma-shaped nuclei predominate
- Nuclei have tapered, pointed or rounded ends
- Preserved cells often have thin bipolar cytoplasmic processes
- Variable presence of pleomorphic and/or multinucleated tumour cells
- Nuclei hyperchromatic, often with prominent nucleoli
- Heterotopic tissue rarely found

Epithelioid MPNST

- Epithelioid MPNST features polygonal or rounded epithel-like tumour cells

Differential diagnosis

- Ancient neurilemoma
- Cellular schwannoma
- Leiomyosarcoma
- Synovial sarcoma
- Fibrosarcoma
- Pleomorphic sarcoma of another lineage
- Carcinoma metastasis (epithelioid MPNST)

Comment

The majority of MPNST are diagnosed as spindle cell sarcoma or pleomorphic sarcoma with FNA. The cellular features may suggest MPNST but a diagnosis may be difficult, even with the help of adjunctive methods. IC may be of diagnostic help if S-100 protein is positive. The positivity in MPNST is typically focal, extensive staining favours a cellular schwannoma. Negative staining with desmin, SMA and muscle-specific actin excludes smooth muscle tumours and negative staining with cytokeratin, EMA and CD99 excludes most synovial sarcoma.

EM may indicate a Schwann cell origin. Low-grade MPNST may be misinterpreted as a neurilemoma. Although the cellular pleomorphism may be marked in ancient neurilemoma, the large atypical, bizarre cells are not numerous and usually the smears contain areas typical of benign neurilemoma.

Malignant Granular Cell Tumour

Malignant granular cell tumours are extremely rare. Histopathological criteria of malignancy have been proposed, but some malignant granular cell tumours cannot be distinguished from benign ones. Features which have been considered to suggest malignancy are necrosis, a predominance of spindly tumour cells, cellular pleomorphism, prominent nucleoli and mitoses.

Vascular Tumours

Vascular tumours comprise a diagnostically difficult group of soft tissue tumours. A substantial number of more or less rare subtypes, benign, borderline and malignant, have been defined clinicopathologically. However, cytological

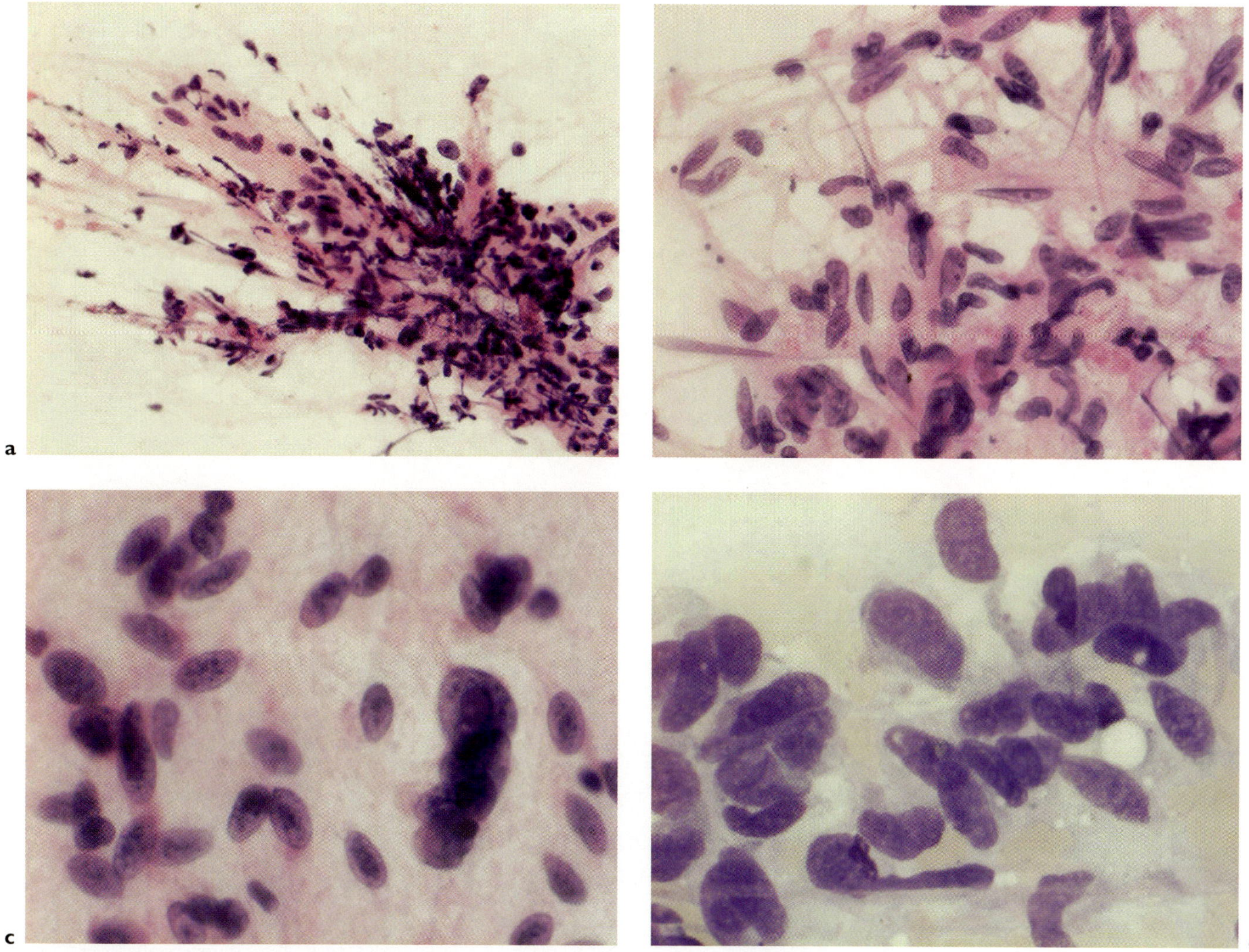

Fig. 52. MPNST. **a** A group of loosely cohesive, moderately atypical cells with a fibrillary background. HE. Low magnification. **b** Spindle-shaped cells with elongated nuclei with pointed ends or comma-shaped. Note fibrillary background. HE. Medium magnification. **c** Variable nuclear pleomorphism. HE. High magnification. **d** Nuclei in MPNST may have rounded ends similar to leiomyosarcoma. MGG. High magnification.

criteria for diagnosis are lacking or incomplete in most types. Many variants have so far not been described and for others only individual case reports have been published.

Of the benign varieties, haemangioma (subcutaneous and intramuscular) is the one most often referred for FNA. It has been suggested that cytological criteria for a confident diagnosis of haemangioma may be present in smears [97] but in our experience, a suggested diagnosis of haemangioma is in the majority of cases an exclusion diagnosis supplemented by clinical and radiographic findings.

Cytological features of haemangioma (fig. 53a, b)

Haemorrhagic aspirates; the syringe may partially fill with blood, even without aspiration

Paucicellular smears

Small runs or groups of spindly cells in variable, often low numbers

Intact cells have elongated nuclei with pointed ends and thin cytoplasmic processes

Variable presence of histiocytes, including siderophages

Variable presence of fragments of adipose tissue with or without vessel fragments

Differential diagnosis

Any benign soft tissue tumour, which is richly vascularized and predominantly composed of spindle cells

Benign adipose tumours

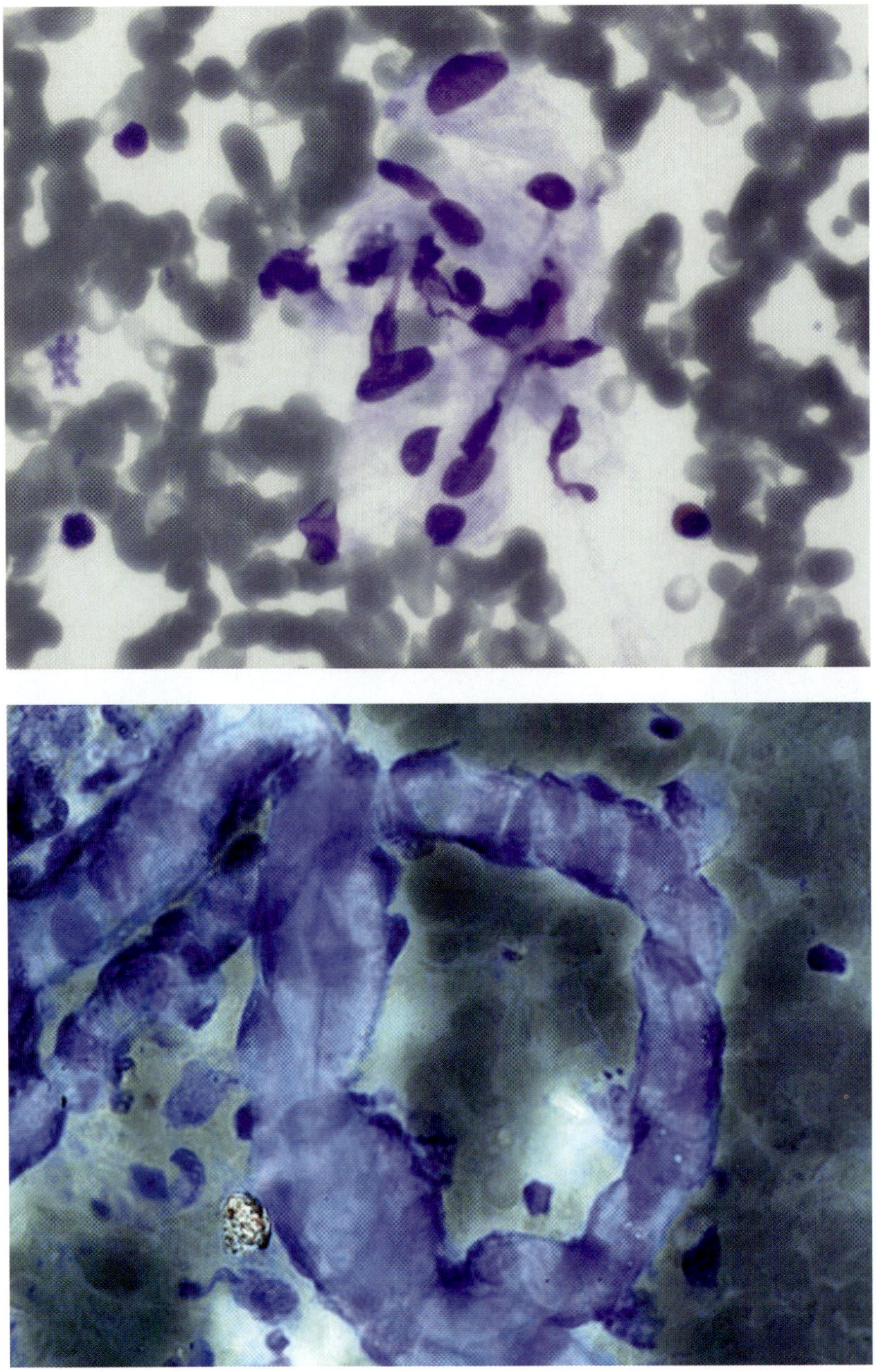

a

b

Fig. 53. Haemangioma. **a** A small group of uniform spindly cells. MGG. Medium magnification. **b** Capillary vessel fragments, an unusual finding in smears from haemangioma. MGG. High magnification. Neither **a** nor **b** are diagnostic of haemangioma per se.

Comment

A suggested diagnosis of haemangioma is based on the combined evaluation of the clinical investigation (haemangioma in a limb usually increases in size during exercise and decreases at rest), MRI imaging features, and the cytological findings. A source for misinterpretation is the frequent presence of adipose tissue in haemangioma. The best way to clinch a diagnosis of haemangioma is to prove that the spindle cells are endothelial cells. As CD34 is positive in a number of non-vascular spindle cell tumours, other endothelial cell markers such as CD31 and factor VIII must be applied.

Malignant Tumours

Angiosarcoma

Angiosarcoma is typically a cutaneous tumour, less than 20% are diagnosed in the deep soft tissues.

Histopathology

Differentiated tumours are made up of irregular vascular channels lined by endothelial cells of varying shapes, showing pleomorphism and nuclear atypia. Clusters of tumour cells are often multilayered and cell tufts and papillary extensions are common. Obvious vascular channels may be difficult to find in poorly differentiated angiosarcoma. Intracytoplasmic vacuoles containing individual or small groups of erythrocytes may be the only sign indicating a vasoformative tumour. A subset of angiosarcoma has large and epithelioid tumour cells.

The majority of angiosarcomas stain for CD31, less often for CD34, and only occasionally do the tumor cells stain positive for factor VIII. Up to half of epithelioid angiosarcomas stain for cytokeratin and some for EMA. Electron-microscopic examination may demonstrate endothelial differentiation (Weibel-Palade bodies, pinocytosis and external laminae).

As in histological sections, the cellular composition of angiosarcoma is very variable in smears including atypical spindle cells, rounded and polygonal cells, binucleated cells, variable chromatin texture and nucleolar size, and a variable amount of cytoplasm. Three relatively large series describing the cytological features of angiosarcoma have been published [47–49].

Cytological features of angiosarcoma (fig. 54a–e)

- Variable cell yield
- More or less haemorrhagic aspirates
- Dispersed cells, cell groups and cell aggregates
- Infrequently acinar-like structures with or without central erythrocytes
- A pleomorphic cell population is more common than a predominant spindle cell population
- Epithelial-like cells
- Signet-ring-like cells with individual erythrocytes within a cytoplasmic vacuole
- Variable nuclear atypia

Differential diagnosis

- Spindle cell sarcoma of various lines of differentiation
- Pleomorphic sarcoma of various lines of differentiation
- Malignant melanoma
- Metastatic carcinoma

Comment

The cell population of most angiosarcomas is recognized as malignant in smears. A specific diagnosis of angiosarcoma, based on the examination of routinely stained material, is not often possible. Those cases where vasoformative structures in the form of small acinar-like formations with central erythrocytes or vacuolated cells with individual erythrocytes are found are an exception. As evident from the cytopathological features, one very important pitfall is to mistake an angiosarcoma (especially epithelioid angiosarcoma) for a metastatic carcinoma.

A reliable type-specific diagnosis requires an immunocytochemical investigation with CD31 and factor VIII besides CD34. The demonstration of cytoplasmic Weibel-Palade bodies by EM is yet another method to confirm the endothelial origin of the tumour cells.

Perivascular Tumours

Glomus tumour and haemangiopericytoma are considered to be examples of perivascular tumours. A diagnosis of haemangiopericytoma of the deep soft tissues, pelvic region and retroperitoneum can occasionally be suggested by FNA. The concept that all haemangiopericytomas are examples of pericytic tumours has, however, been debated. It has been suggested that the sinonasal haemangiopericytoma is composed of cells resembling pericytes while a pericytic origin has not been documented in haemangiopericytoma of soft tissues and retroperitoneum. Several other soft tissue tumours may have a haemangiopericytoma-like microscopic pattern, especially the vascular architecture. Among the soft tissue tumours with a haemangiopericytoma-like vascular pattern the most important the cytopathologist should consider are synovial sarcoma and solitary fibrous tumour [98, 99].

Glomus Tumour

Glomus tumours are generally small tumours, usually less than 1 cm. The most common site is the subungual region of the fingers followed by other parts of the extremities, mostly wrist and foot. Glomus tumours may, however, appear in almost every part of the body. Patients are usually young to middle-aged adults. Characteristically the glomus tumours are painful; radiating paroxysmal pain and cold intolerance are common. These tumours are rare targets for FNA since the most common small painful subungual tumours are almost never referred for needling. Individual case reports of the cytomorphology of glomus tumours have been published [100].

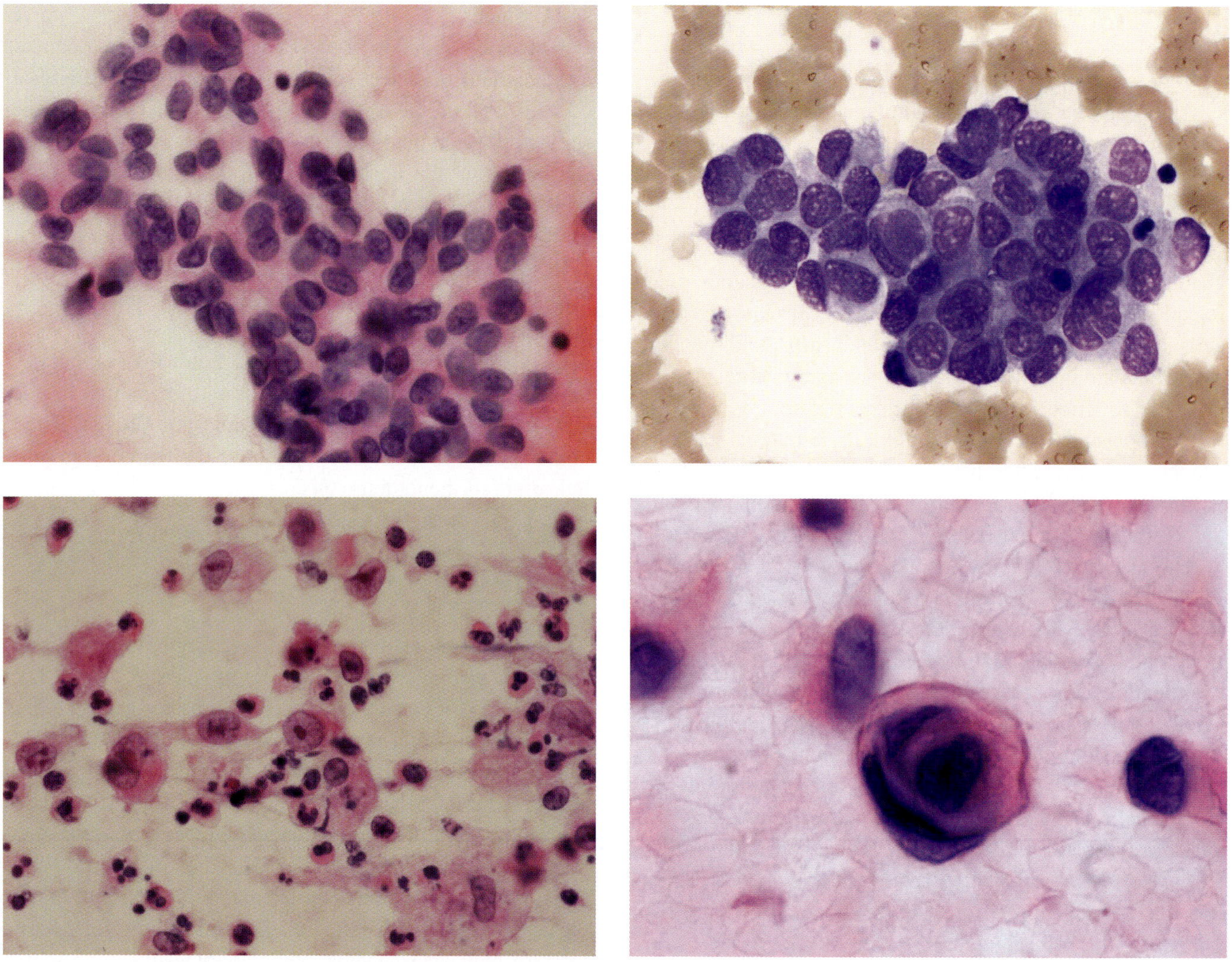

a b c d

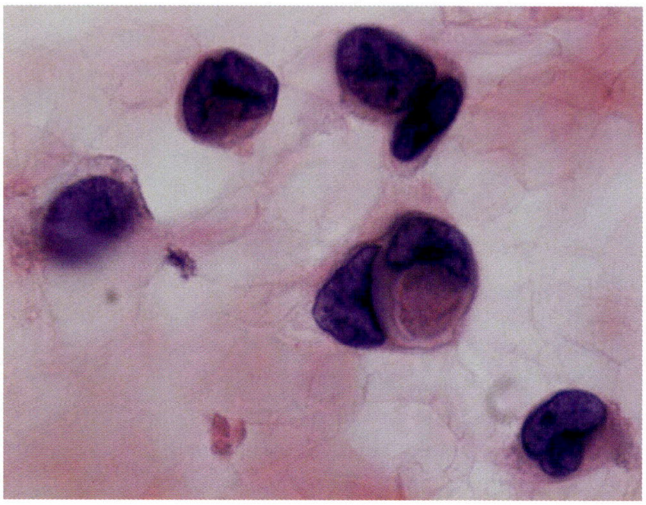

e

Fig. 54. Angiosarcoma. The cytological patterns of angiosarcoma in FNA smears are variable. **a** A cluster of epithelial-like cells showing mild to moderate nuclear atypia. HE. Medium magnification. **b** An epithelial-like cluster of tightly crowded cells. Note nuclear moulding. MGG. Medium magnification. **c** A rather poor yield of dispersed tumour cells with abundant cytoplasm and rounded atypical nuclei with prominent nucleoli. HE. Medium magnification. **d**, **e** Tumour cells from a case of epithelioid angiosarcoma. Note vacuolated cell in **e**. HE. High magnification.

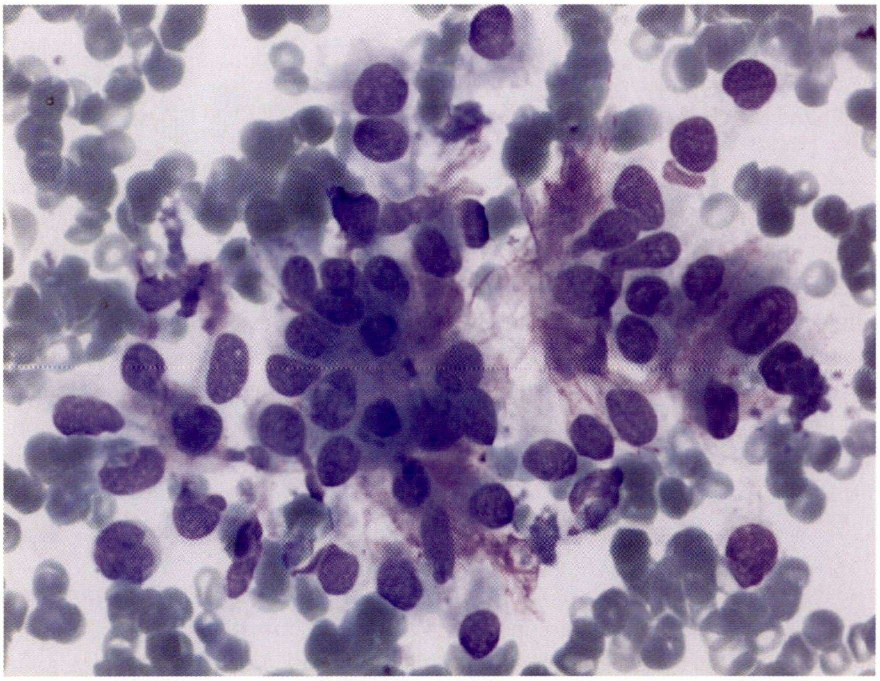

a

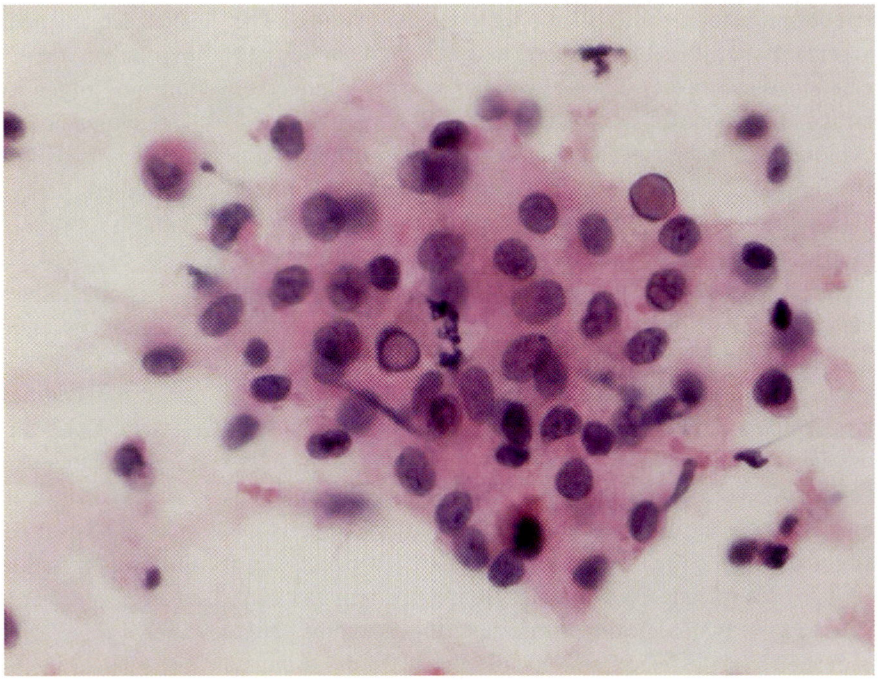

b

Fig. 55. Glomus tumour. **a** A cluster of cells separated by a myxoid fibrillary matrix. MGG Medium magnification. **b** The tumour cells have rounded, bland nuclei with abundant, poorly defined cytoplasm. HE. Medium magnification.

Histopathology

Glomus tumours are composed of rounded uniform cells with rounded uniform nuclei. They form sheets or clusters surrounding blood vessels. The stroma is hyalinized or myxoid. The cells stain for SMA and vimentin and in some tumours focally for desmin.

Cytological features of glomus tumour (fig. 55a, b)

Variable yield, often haemorrhagic aspirates
Dispersed cells and cell clusters
Variable amount of myxoid fibrillary background matrix
The lesional cells are of medium size with poorly defined cytoplasmic borders and rounded or ovoid bland nuclei with inconspicuous nucleoli

Differential diagnosis
Angiomyoma
Epithelioid vascular neoplasms
Epithelial tumours

Comment

Needling of glomus tumours is, as in the case of neurilemoma and angiomyoma, most often painful. In the common sites such as the extremities, the diagnosis is facilitated by clinical findings. In other sites glomus tumours may be difficult to distinguish from epithelial tumours and epithelioid vascular neoplasms. IC is of diagnostic help. Negative staining for cytokeratins and endothelial cell markers such as CD31 and CD34 together with positive staining for SMA suggests the diagnosis.

Haemangiopericytoma of Soft Tissue

Histopathology

These are usually macroscopically well-circumscribed tumours. Cystic degeneration, haemorrhagic areas and necrosis may be found. The typical microscopic pattern consists of numerous, thin-walled often branching vessels. The vascular pattern has been likened to stag horns. The tumour cells surrounding the vessels are often randomly arranged or arranged in bundles or sheets. The cells have elongated, ovoid or rounded nuclei and show a rather uniform chromatin structure. The cell margins are indistinct and the mitotic activity is variable. Tumour cell necrosis, a high rate of mitoses and the presence of pleomorphic, atypical cells are features indicative of malignancy. However, tumours with bland cells and low mitotic activity may also metastasize. The diagnosis of soft tissue haemangiopericytoma is considered a diagnosis of exclusion when other soft tissue tumours with a similar architecture have been ruled out. In about half of the haemangiopericytomas tested, the tumour cells, besides the endothelial cells, stain for CD34. Desmin, actin and CD99 are negative. Ultrastructurally, the tumour cells are fibroblast-like.

Our files include FNA samples from a few tumours considered to be histologically proven haemangiosarcomas after exclusion of synovial sarcoma and of solitary fibrous tumour.

Cytological features of haemangiopericytoma (fig. 56a–c)
Often haemorrhagic aspirates, variable cellularity
Dispersed cells and cellular small tissue fragments
Many stripped nuclei
A branching vascular network seen in tissue fragments
Isolated branching vessel fragments with tumour cells clustered on the vessel walls found occasionally
Small- to medium-sized tumour cells with elongated, ovoid or rounded bland nuclei
Short bipolar cytoplasmic processes in intact individual cells

Differential diagnosis
Synovial sarcoma
Solitary fibrous tumour

Comment

The diagnosis of haemangiopericytoma is as difficult in FNA smears as in histological sections. It is mandatory to exclude synovial sarcoma, which may have similar features in routinely stained smears. Due to the common CD34 positivity in both solitary fibrous tumour and haemangiopericytoma, the distinction between these two tumours is sometimes not possible cytologically.

Paraganglionic Tumours

Paraganglionic tumours are neuroendocrine tumours of neural crest origin associated with the autonomic ganglia. The head and neck region (carotid body, vagal body, glomus jugulare), mediastinum (aortic body) and retroperitoneum (organs of Zuckerkandl) are the sites of origin. The cytopathologist is mainly involved in the diagnosis of carotid body paraganglioma. Mediastinal and retroperitoneal paragangliomas are infrequently investigated with FNA.

Histopathology

Paragangliomas have variable morphological features. The most characteristic pattern is tumour cells arranged in small rounded nests (zell ballen) surrounded by thin-walled vessels. Cords or ribbons, rosette-like or gland-like structures are other patterns. The tumour cells are mainly rounded or polygonal, epithelioid-like with abundant cytoplasm, but spindle-shaped cells also occur. Anisokaryosis varies: a not uncommon finding is scattered large, atypical cells within an otherwise rather uniform cell population. The cytoplasm is finely granular, but may be vacuolated or may contain intranuclear inclusions. The tumour cells stain positively for NSE and chromogranin and synaptophysin can be demonstrated in most tumours. The most important ultrastructural finding is the presence of small dense-core granules, measuring 100–200 nm in diameter.

Diagnostic criteria for malignancy in paraganglioma are a debated issue. High mitotic activity, necrosis, marked pleomorphism and vascular invasion have been proposed as malignant features by some while others consider that metastatic spread is the only reliable sign of malignancy.

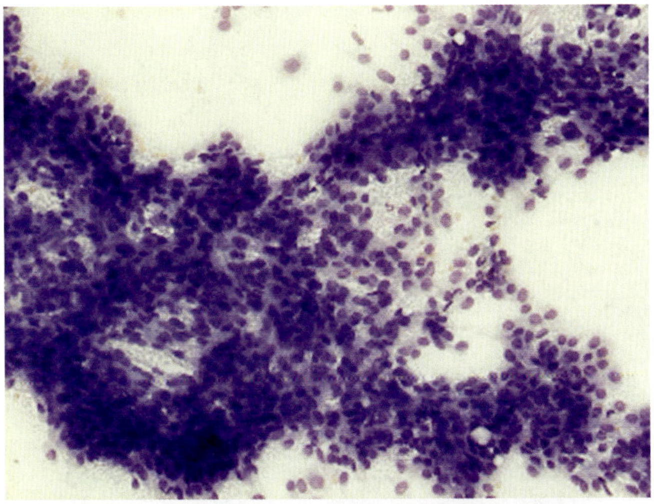

a

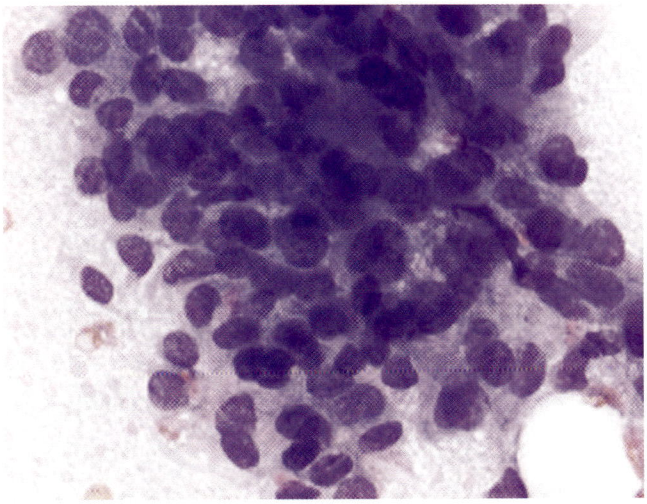

b

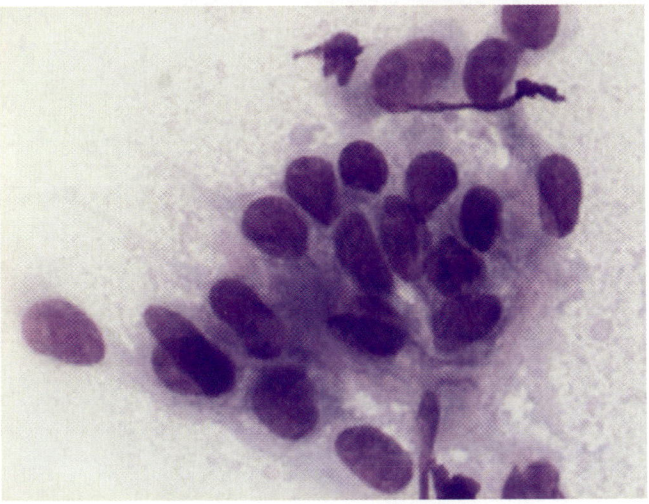

c

Fig. 56. Malignant haemangiopericytoma. **a** Branching highly cellular tissue fragments associated with dispersed cells. Synovial sarcoma may have the same appearance under low power. MGG. Low magnification. **b**, **c** The tumour cells are small to medium-sized with ovoid or rounded bland nuclei. MGG. High magnification.

Of all paragangliomas, the cytological features of carotid body paraganglioma (chemodectoma) have been most thoroughly investigated [101–103].

Cytological features of paraganglioma (fig. 57a, b)

- Individual cells and clusters of loosely cohesive cells
- Occasional gland-like or follicle-like groupings
- Mainly rounded or polygonal epithelioid-like cells with rather abundant cytoplasm
- Moderate cellular and nuclear pleomorphism
- Scattered large cells with large, hyperchromatic nuclei
- Red cytoplasmic granularity (MGG), similar to that of medullary thyroid carcinoma

Differential diagnosis

- Medullary thyroid carcinoma
- Adenocarcinoma

Comment

Most tumours biopsied with FNA are carotid body paragangliomas in the neck. The main differential diagnosis in this site is medullary carcinoma of the thyroid.

Malignant Tumours

Malignant Paraganglioma

Cytological features favouring malignancy have not been described. In histological sections, necrosis and mitotic activity are probably the most useful of the criteria that have been suggested to indicate malignancy.

Extragastrointestinal Stromal Tumours

Tumours with a phenotype similar to gastrointestinal stromal tumours (GISTs) may arise in the omentum, mesentery

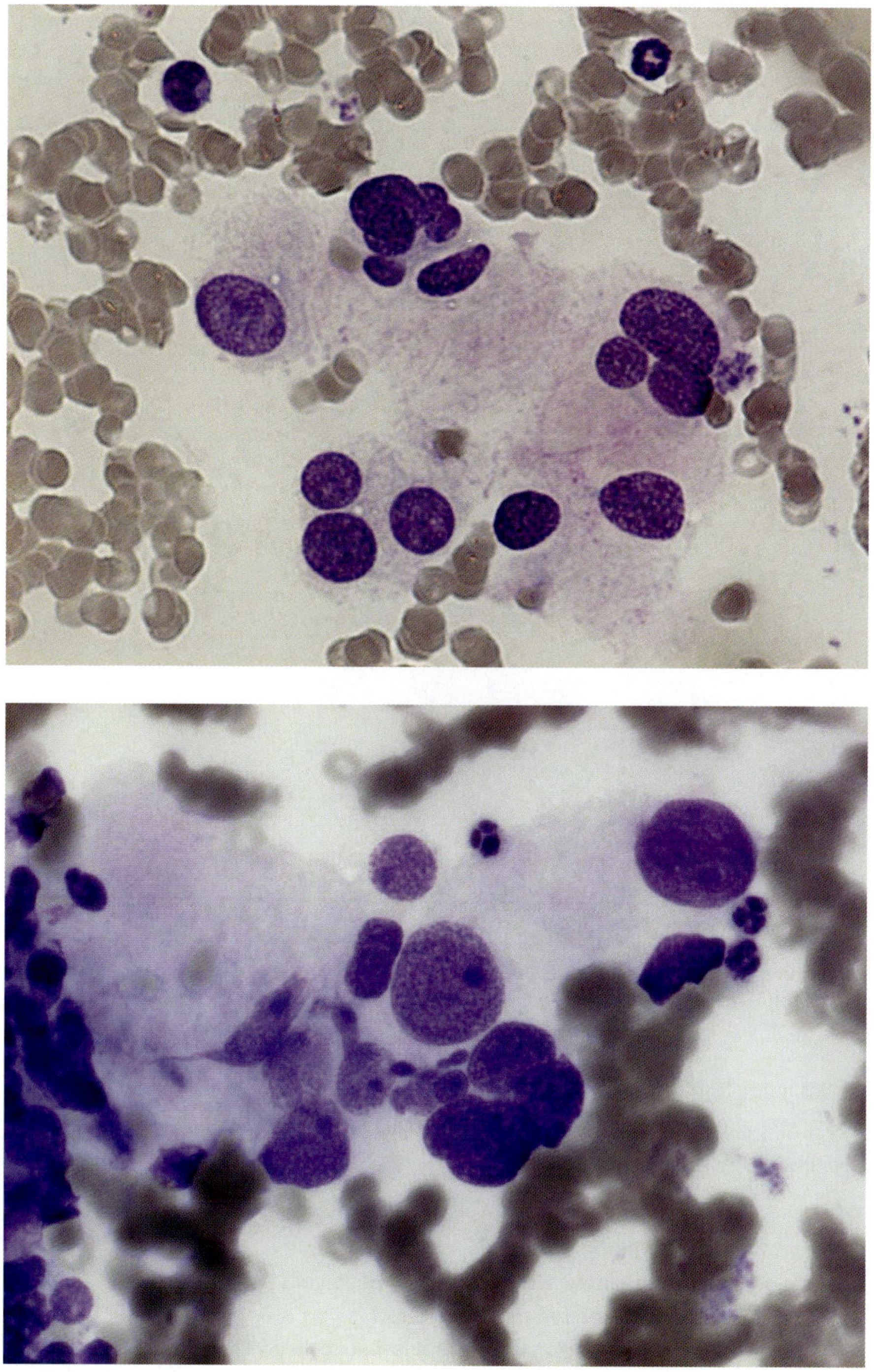

a

b

Fig. 57. Paraganglioma. **a** A cluster of poorly cohesive cells. Abundant, faintly granular cytoplasm and moderate anisokaryosis. MGG. Medium magnification. **b** Nuclear pleomorphism may be prominent. MGG. Medium magnification.

or in the retroperitoneum. They are uncommon but are important differential diagnostic considerations versus other mesenchymal tumours in those sites.

Histopathology

GISTs have a very variable morphology but usually one of two patterns dominate: spindle cell and epithelioid. The two patterns may coexist in some tumours. The epithelioid population is composed of round cells of varying sizes with eosinophilic cytoplasm and rounded nuclei. Cytoplasmic vacuolation may be seen; at times cells resembling signet ring cells are observed. The epithelioid cells are mostly arranged in groups or nests in a collagenous or myxoid stroma. The spindle cell population consists of fusiform cells with ovoid nuclei. The cells are arranged in fascicular bundles or in a vaguely storiform pattern. Nuclear palisading is occasionally seen.

The tumours may be hypercellular and show marked cellular atypia including multinucleated large tumour cells. The main immunohistochemical profile is a positive reaction for c-kit (CD117) and CD34. CD117 is positive in almost all cases and CD34 in about 50%. Some GISTs express SMA but desmin is negative.

Ultrastructurally the tumour cells may display neural as well as smooth muscle features. GISTs often express activity mutations of the c-*kit* gene.

During recent years several articles on FNA of GISTs have been published [104–106].

With FNA, as with histopathological evaluation, two main patterns are identified: the spindle cell type and epithelioid type.

Cytological features of extragastrointestinal stromal tumour, spindle cell type (fig. 58a–d)

- Cellular smears
- Cohesive clusters or fascicles of tightly packed cells
- Stripped nuclei common
- Nuclei spindly, ovoid, comma-shaped or cigar-shaped with finely granular chromatin
- Scanty cytoplasm, occasionally cytoplasmic processes
- Cytoplasmic vacuoles occasionally seen

Cytological features of extragastrointestinal stromal tumour, epithelioid type (fig. 59a, b)

- Both dispersed cells and cells in groups or clusters
- Rounded, polygonal or ovoid cells with relatively abundant cytoplasm
- Rounded or ovoid nuclei
- Cytoplasmic vacuolation common

Differential diagnosis

- Leiomyosarcoma
- Peripheral nerve sheath tumours
- Carcinoma

Comment

It is very difficult or almost impossible to confidently distinguish GIST from smooth muscle and peripheral nerve sheath tumours in routinely stained smears. The diagnosis of GIST in fine needle aspirates should be based on the combined evaluation of routinely stained smears and IC (double positivity of CD117 and CD34 is an important diagnostic sign). Mutational analysis of the c-*kit* gene in FNA aspirates has been described [106].

Primitive Neuroectodermal Tumours

Among the tumours categorized as PNET, the ones most important to the cytopathologist are the neuroblastoma and the related ganglioneuroblastoma and ganglioneuroma, and the extraskeletal tumours of the ES/PNET family. Tumours of the ES/PNET family have a variable morphology and immunophenotype. The common denominator is their cytogenetic aberration, t(11;22)(q24;q12). Several investigators have found this translocation or variants thereof, also involving 22q12 (the EWS gene) in about 90% of tumours investigated

Neuroblastoma

Neuroblastoma is the most common extracranial solid malignant tumour in children. Ninety percent are diagnosed before the age of 5 years. As neuroblastoma and ganglioneuroblastoma originate in symphathetic ganglia, they are mostly found in a paramedline position. The retroperitoneum is the most frequent site followed by the mediastinum and the sacral region. Not infrequently, the initial diagnosis of a neuroblastoma is made with FNA of a metastatic deposit. Metastases are most commonly found in bone, lymph nodes, liver and skin.

Histopathology

The neuroblastoma is a typical example of the 'small round cell tumour' of childhood. Neuroblastomas are composed of ill-defined lobules of tumour cells bordered by thin fibrovascular septa. The tumour cells have rounded or irregular nuclei with finely granular, clumped chromatin. Nucleoli are inconspicuous. There is a variable amount of intercellular fibrillary material (neuropil) of neuritic cell processes. Rosette-like structures with a central core of fibrillary material are a typical feature (Homer-Wright rosettes). In undifferentiated neuroblastoma the fibrillary matrix may be missing while large ganglion cell-like cells are present in more mature tumours. Positive immunostaining for NSE, chromogranin and synaptophysin is a common finding, but staining for chromogranin and synaptophysin may be negative in undifferentiated tumours. Ultrastructurally, neuritic processes with neurotubules and uniform dense-core granules are characteristic features. The cytological features of neuroblastoma have been studied in several cases [45, 46].

Cytological features of neuroblastoma (fig. 60a–d)

- Most commonly a cell-rich yield
- Cells both in clusters or groups and dispersed
- Cells often embedded in a fibrillary background

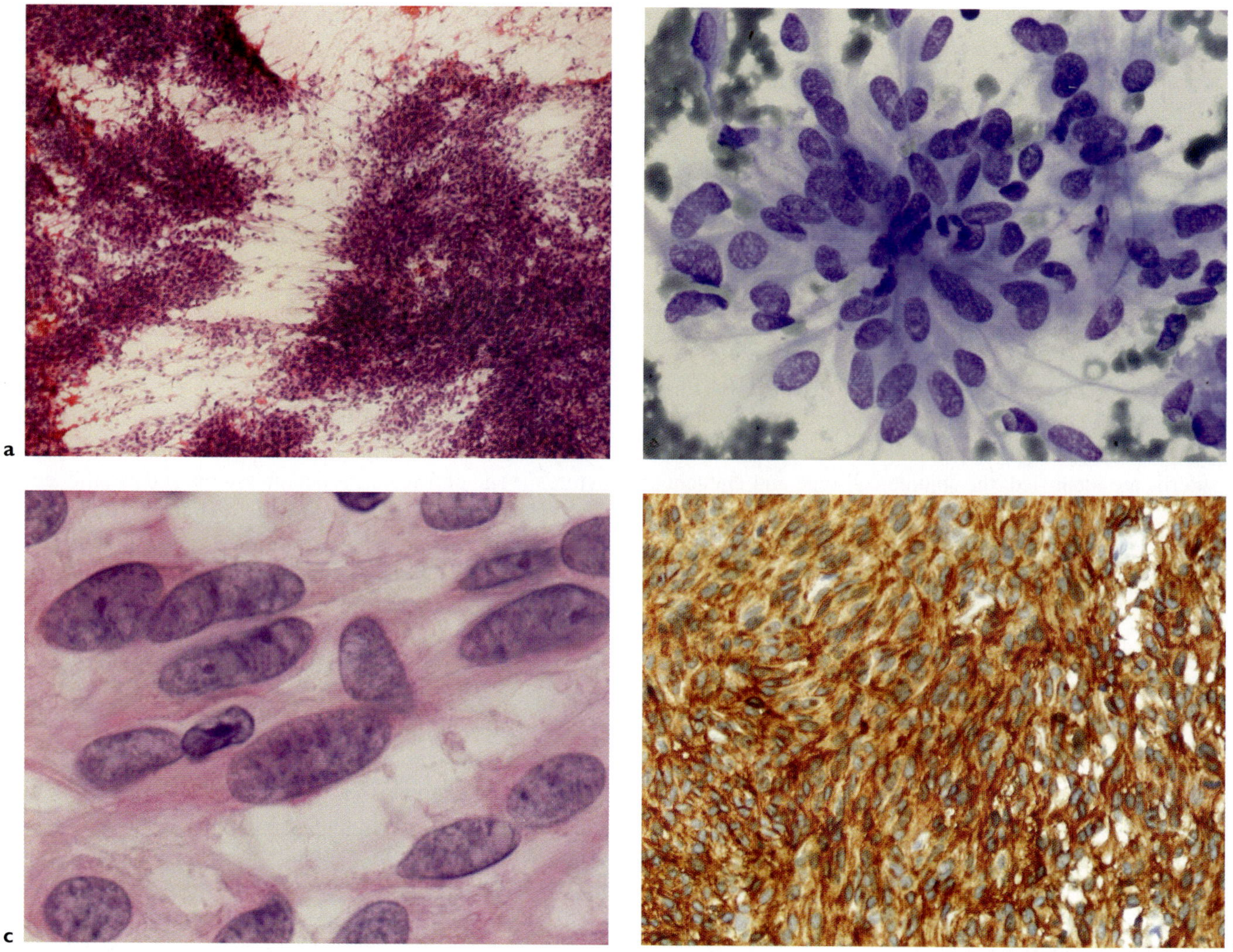

Fig. 58. Extragastrointestinal stromal tumour, spindle cell type. **a** Under low power magnification there are both cellular tissue fragments and dispersed cells. HE. Low magnification. **b** Nuclei are spindle-shaped, ovoid or comma-shaped with bland chromatin. MGG. High magnification. **c** The spindle-shaped nuclei may be difficult to distinguish from smooth muscle cell nuclei. HE, oil. **d** Positive staining with CD117 is necessary to confirm the diagnosis of extragastrointestinal stromal tumour. CD117 on cell block preparation.

Cells often arranged in an Indian file pattern or in small moulded clusters
Variable presence of rosette-like structures with a central fibrillary core
Tumour cells have irregular, hyperchromatic nuclei and uni- or bipolar cytoplasm with slender processes
Cells often have anastomosing cytoplasmic processes
Depending on the degree of differentiation there is a variable presence of triangular or polyhedral ganglion cell-like cells with abundant cytoplasm and rounded nucleolated eccentric nuclei

Differential diagnosis

Alveolar rhabdomyosarcoma
ES/PNET family of tumours
Precursor lymphoma/acute lymphoblastic leukaemia
Wilms' tumour

Comment

In a study of 19 neuroblastomas from our files, we found the most common combination of cytological features to be neuropil, moulded clusters and anastomosing thin cytoplasmic processes [46]. Rosettes and cytoplasmic processes are absent or rare in undifferentiated or poorly differentiated neuroblastoma.

IC and EM are helpful in the diagnosis. NSE staining may be focally positive and chromogranin and synaptophysin negative in undifferentiated neuroblastoma.

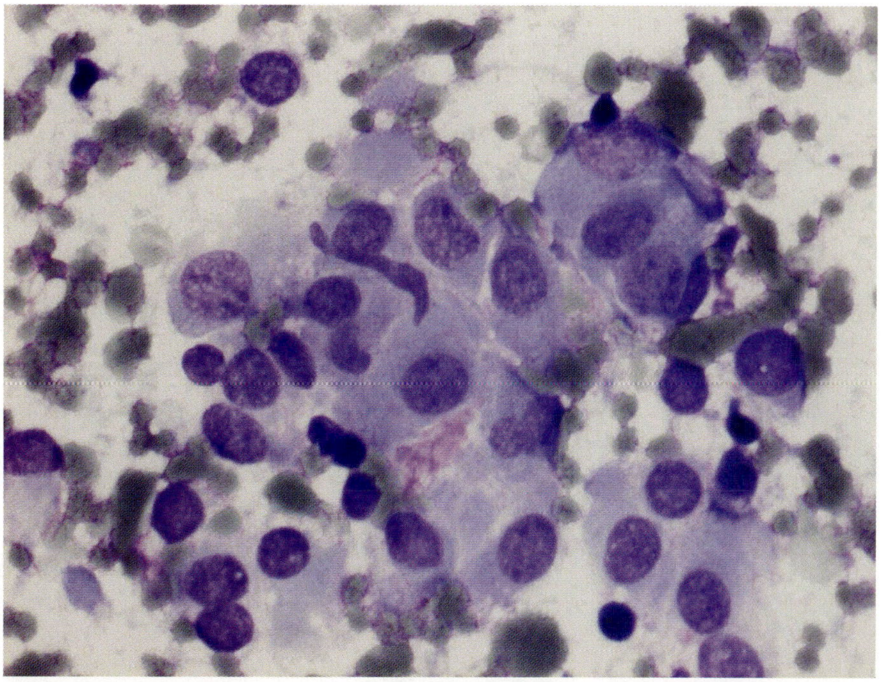

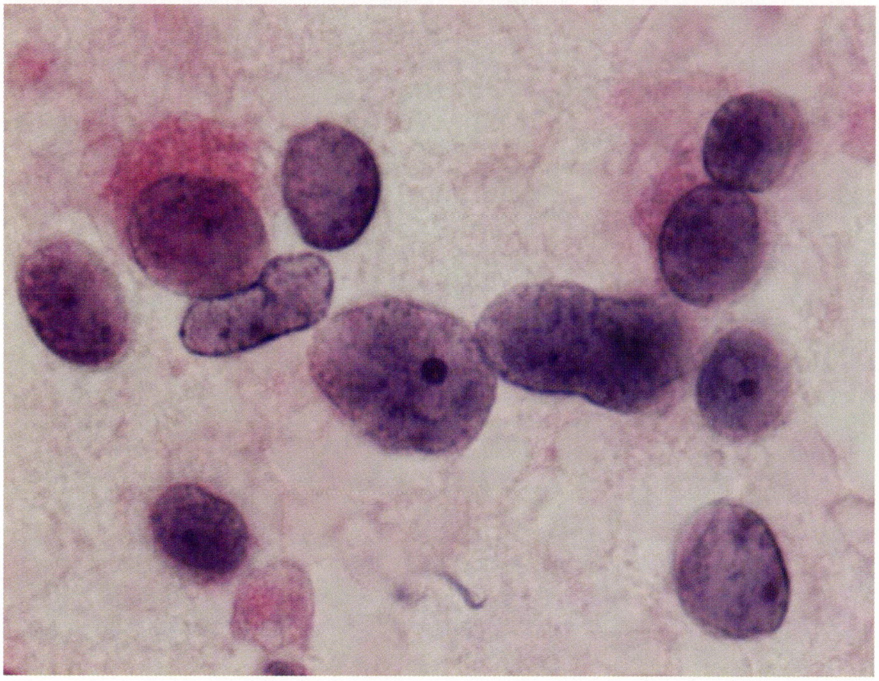

Fig. 59. Extragastrointestinal stromal tumour, round cell type. **a** A cluster of epithelial-like rounded cells with relatively abundant cytoplasm and rounded nuclei. MGG. Medium magnification. **b** Cells from round cell type of GIST. HE, oil.

Ganglioneuroblastoma

Ganglioneuroblastoma is characterized by the presence of differentiating ganglion cells besides the typical small cells [107].

Ganglioneuroma

There are few reports on the cytopathology of ganglioneuroma in FNA samples [107]. The typical finding is a double cell population of large ganglion cells and neurilemoma-like tissue fragments (fig. 61a–c).

ES/PNET Family of Tumours

The majority of patients are adolescents or young adults. The most common sites are the extremities and the chest wall but tumours have been reported arising in lung, genital organs, kidney and subcutis.

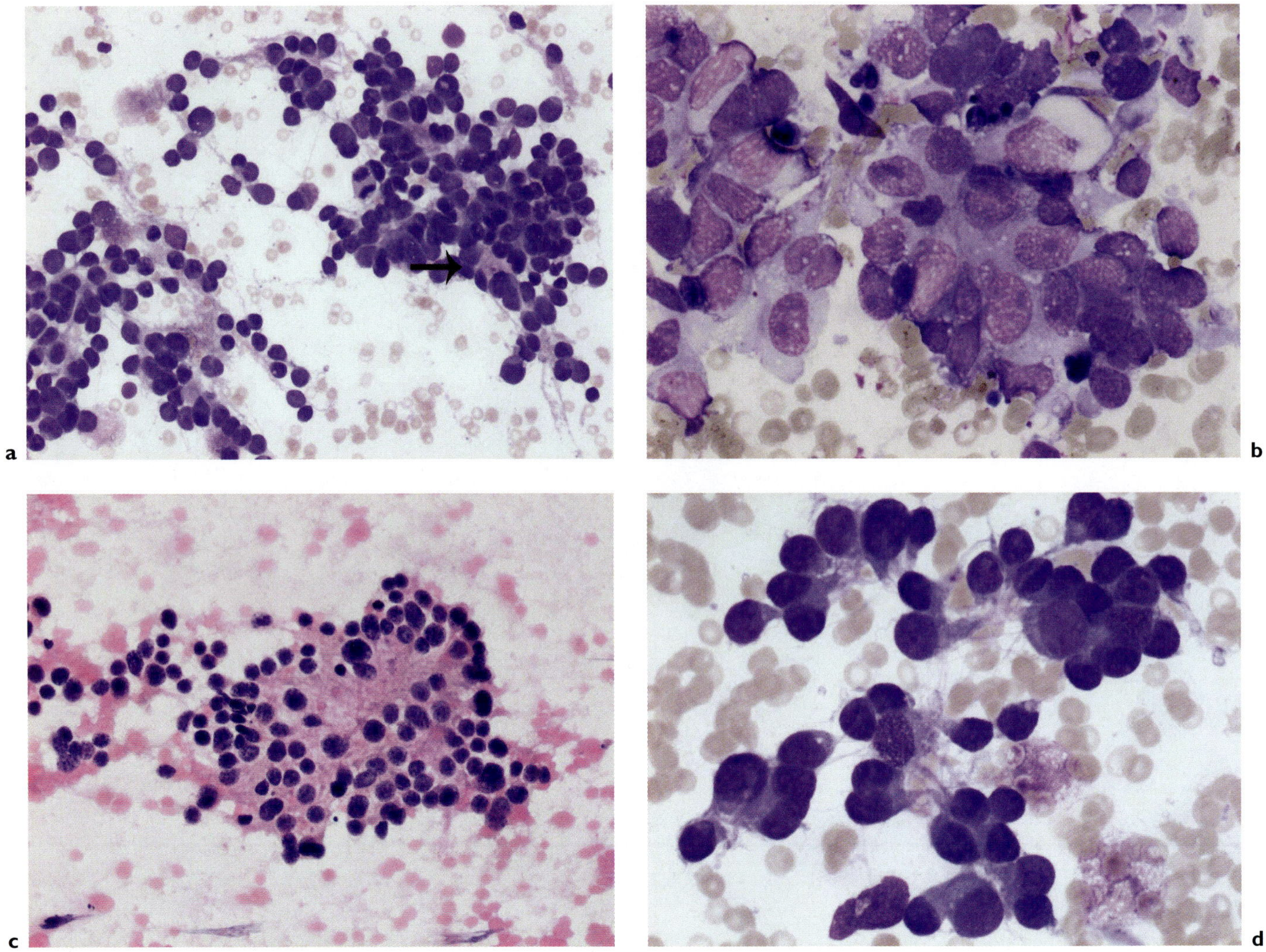

Fig. 60. Neuroblastoma. **a** A highly cellular smear of clustered and dispersed cells. Note rosette-like structure (arrow). MGG. Low magnification. **b** Neuroblastoma cells in smears are often arranged in an Indian file pattern and/or in moulded clusters. MGG. High magnification. **c** A typical rosette-like structure with central neuropil. HE. Medium magnification. **d** The tumour cells often have thin cytoplasmic processes, connecting one cell to another. MGG. High magnification.

Histopathology

The histological features of these tumours vary with the degree of neuroectodermal differentiation. However, a lobular or trabecular pattern with richly vascularized fibrous septa is the most common. Classic ES cells (the least differentiated) have a pale cytoplasm and rounded or ovoid bland nuclei with finely granular chromatin and inconspicuous nucleoli. In more differentiated tumours (PNET) the cellular pleomorphism may be more marked, the nuclear chromatin coarser and the nucleoli prominent. Rosettes with a fibrillary centre and perivascular pseudorosettes may be numerous. The so-called 'atypical ES' is characterized by larger cells and more prominent anisocytosis and anisokaryosis than the classic ES. Cytoplasmic glycogen is typically found in ES, less so in PNET. Immunohistochemically, a positive staining for CD99 is common to all variants. In addition, there is a spectrum from only vimentin positivity (classic ES) to the presence of various neuroectodermal antibodies such as NSA, chromogranin and synaptophysin (PNET). Ultrastructurally, there is, as with immunohistochemical stainings, a spectrum of features, depending on the differentiation: a paucity of organelles and large glycogen deposits in ES, an increasing presence of neurotubules and neurosecretory granules and cell processes in PNET. The cytology of classic ES as well as atypical ES and PNET has been quite extensively studied in individual cases and series [108–113].

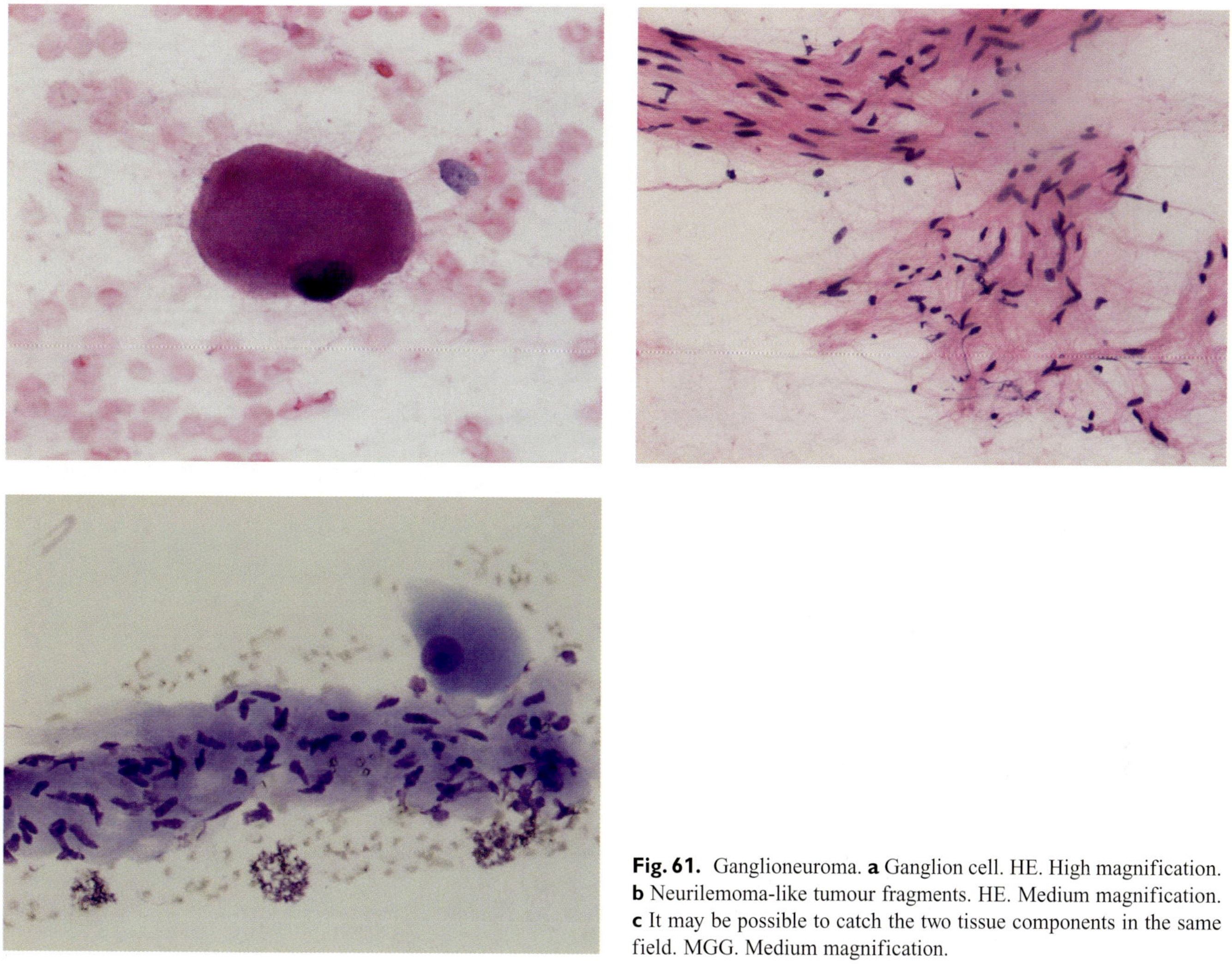

Fig. 61. Ganglioneuroma. **a** Ganglion cell. HE. High magnification. **b** Neurilemoma-like tumour fragments. HE. Medium magnification. **c** It may be possible to catch the two tissue components in the same field. MGG. Medium magnification.

Cytological features of conventional ES (fig. 62a, b)

Highly cellular yield as a rule

Cells both clustered and dispersed

Stripped nuclei and cytoplasmic background common

Double cell population; large cells with abundant fragile cytoplasm with vacuoles or clear spaces and rounded bland nuclei with inconspicuous nucleoli (large, light cells); small cells with irregular dark nuclei and scanty cytoplasm (small, dark cells); the dark cells are often arranged in small moulded groups within the cell clusters

Cytological features of atypical ES (fig. 63)

Cellular and nuclear pleomorphism more marked than in conventional ES

Typical large light cells less numerous than in conventional ES

Some cells with thin cytoplasmic processes

Rosette-like structures with more or less evident fibrillary centre

Cytological features of peripheral neuroectodermal tumour (fig. 64)

Similar pattern as in atypical ES but numerous cells with cytoplasmic processes

Large light cell minority

Rosette-like structures

Differential diagnosis

Alveolar rhabdomyosarcoma

Neuroblastoma

Precursor lymphoma/acute lymphoblastic leukaemia

Poorly differentiated synovial sarcoma

Desmoplastic small round cell tumour

Comment

Smears from conventional ES are very similar in all cases. Pleomorphism is more marked in PNET, and the cells may be more neuroblastoma-like. The distinction between conventional ES, atypical ES and PNET is not of decisive clinical importance as in most centres all varietes are treated alike.

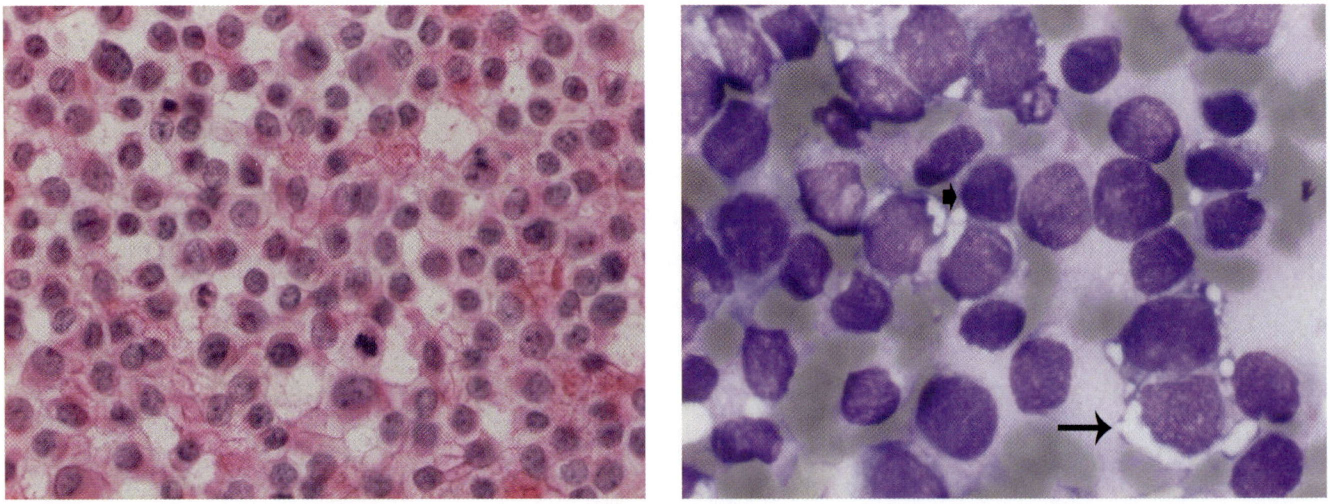

62a 62b

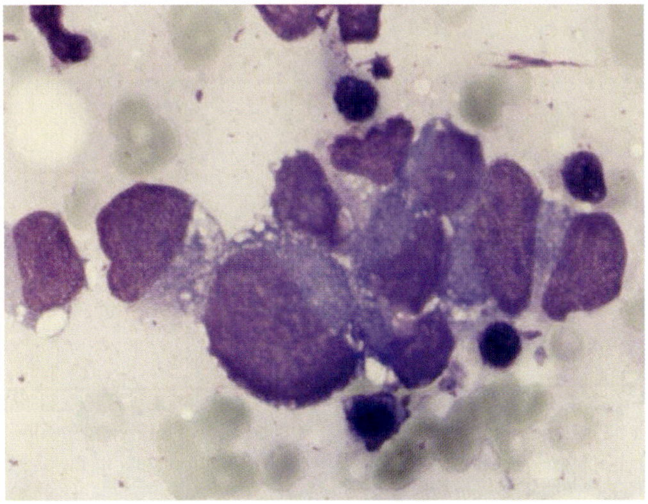

63

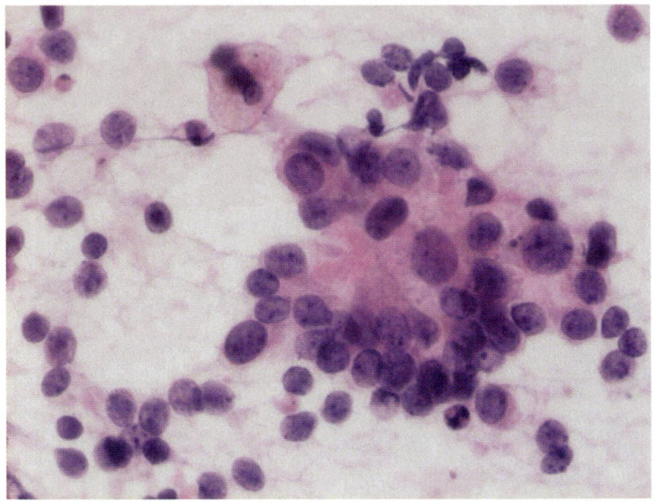

64

Fig. 62. ES/PNET family of tumours. Conventional ES. **a** A cell-rich smear of uniform small rounded cells with rounded nuclei. HE. Low magnification. **b** The two diagnostically important cell types are shown in this field: large light cells (long arrow) and small dark cells (short arrow), best visualized in MGG. MGG. High magnification.

Fig. 63. ES/PNET family of tumours. Atypical ES. The cellular and nuclear pleomorphism is more marked than in conventional ES. MGG. High magnification.

Fig. 64. ES/PNET family of tumours. Rosette-like structure in PNET; structures like this may also be present in atypical ES. HE. High magnification.

The presence of a double cell population has also been described in histological sections. Although the 'small dark cells' are regarded as degenerate cells by most investigators, this feature is an important diagnostic sign in cytological material.

IC and EM are both valuable adjunctive diagnostic methods (fig. 4a, b, 65). CD99 should not be used as a single antibody as it is not specific for the ES/PNET family (table 2).

The cytogenetic/molecular genetic analysis is, in our opinion, the most important ancillary method. The presence of t(11;22)(q24;q12) and/or the fusion transcript between the EWS/FLI1 genes indicate that the tumour in question belongs to the ES/PNET family. FISH of the common EWS breakpoints is another method, well suited for FNA material [66]. It has to be remembered, however, that rearrangements of the EWS gene also occur in desmoplasic small round cell tumour (DSRCT), clear cell sarcoma and myxoid liposarcoma. The two latter tumours present no differential diagnostic problems as their cytology is quite different from that of ES/PNET, but DSRCT may be a diagnostic pitfall in retroperitonal tumours, especially when the yield is poor and the typical double cell population is absent.

FISH should be supplemented with IC in the differential diagnosis between ES/PNET and DSRCT. Due to the polyphenotypic immunoexpression in DSRCT cytokeratins,

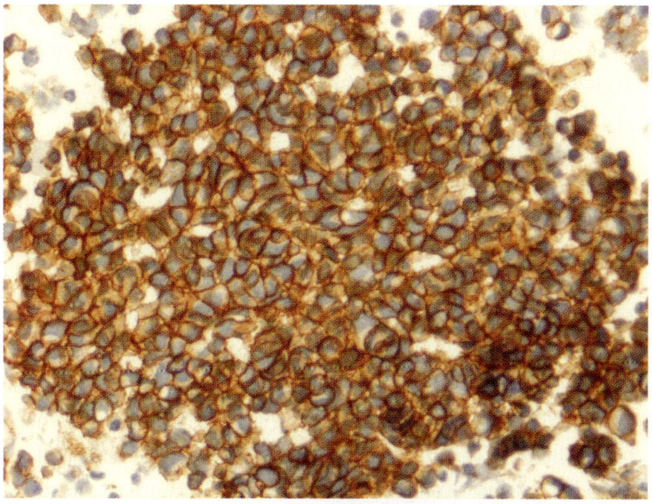

65

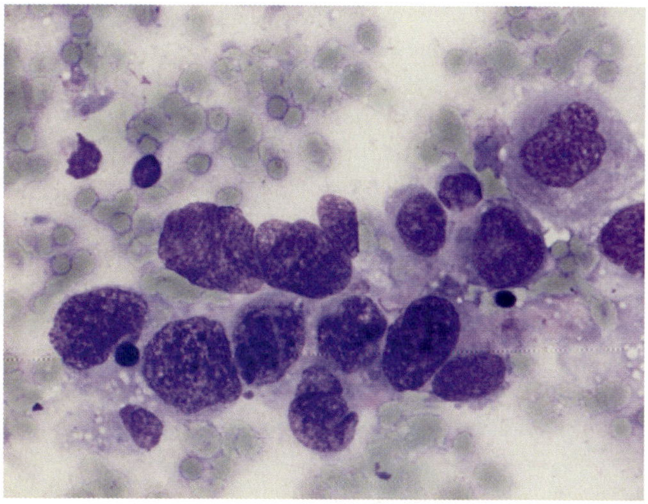

66a

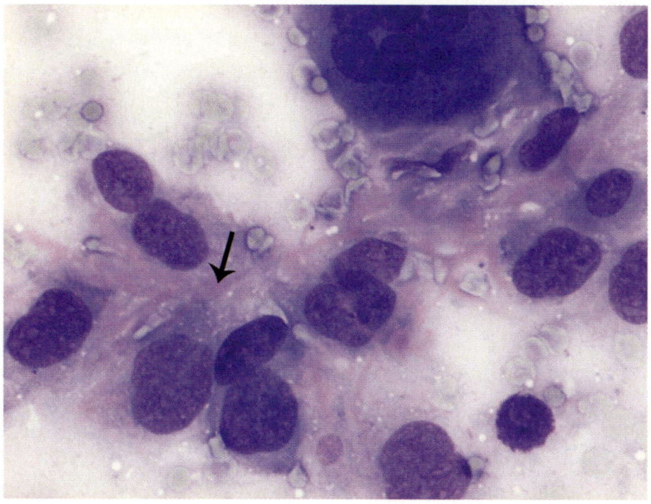

66b

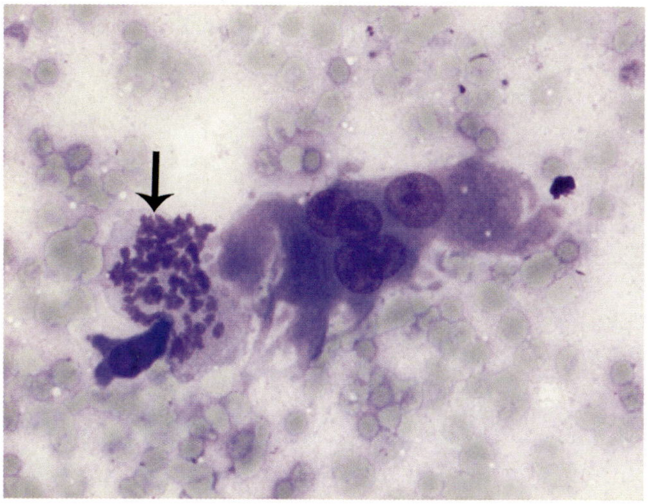

66c

Fig. 65. One criterion common to tumours in the ES/PNET family is positive staining with CD99. CD99 immunostaining on cell block preparation.

Fig. 66. Extraskeletal osteosarcoma. **a** Large, often rounded, pleomorphic tumour cells with rounded nuclei. MGG. Medium magnification. **b** Intercellular strands of osteoid (arrow). MGG. High magnification. **c** Mitotic figures (arrow) are observed in most cases if smears are rich in cells. MGG. Medium magnification.

EMA, desmin and NSE should be part of the antibody panel besides CD99. CD99 has been reported to be focally positive in DSRCT.

In our experience the combined use of electron-microscopic examination and molecular genetic analysis gives the optimal diagnostic information. FNA samples are more suitable for PCR and FISH than for conventional karyotyping [64, 66].

Osseous Tumours

Osteosarcoma of Soft Tissue

Extraskeletal osteosarcoma is a rare sarcoma in middle-aged and old adults. It is extremely rare in children and adolescents. The most frequent site is the legs, less frequently the pelvis, retroperitoneum and arms. Most tumours are deep-seated. Radiographic examination may reveal calcified areas.

Histopathology

Extraskeletal osteosarcoma is a pleomorphic sarcoma resembling the pleomorphic sarcoma of the MFH type. The clue to the diagnosis is the presence of osteoid produced by the tumour cells. The osteoid is usually seen as narrow bands in a lace-like pattern encircling the tumour cells. Extraskeletal osteosarcoma may contain areas of neoplastic cartilage or the tumour cells may be mainly spindle-shaped resembling fibroblastic conventional osteosarcoma.

The cytological features of extraskeletal osteosarcoma have been described in one series [114].

Cytological features of extraskeletal osteosarcoma (fig. 66a–c)

- Variable yield, variably haemorrhagic samples
- Dispersed tumour cells and cell clusters
- Mainly large, rounded, triangular or polygonal highly atypical cells with abundant cytoplasm
- Often eccentric nuclei and variable presence of a paranuclear clear 'hof'
- Bi- and multinucleated tumour cells
- Mitoses, occasionally atypical
- Thin strands of an intercellular matrix often present in cell clusters
- Often admixture of osteoclast-like giant cells
- Atypical spindle cells dominate in the fibroblastic variant

Differential diagnosis

- Other histotypes of pleomorphic soft tissue sarcoma
- Skeletal osteosarcoma

Comment

Most extraskeletal osteosarcoma present as obviously high-grade malignant pleomorphic sarcomas in FNA samples. Exceptions are the rare fibroblastic and small cell variants. The typical extraskeletal osteosarcoma resembles skeletal osteosarcoma in FNA smears. Clinical data and radiographic examinations are of importance to certify that the tumour in question is extraskeletal. In our opinion the intercellular matrix represents osteoid [115]. We have found that staining for alkaline phosphatase as well as osteonectin and osteocalcin are helpful diagnostic adjuncts in the cytological diagnosis of skeletal osteosarcoma [115].

Chapter 5

Tumours of Uncertain or Unknown Origin

Benign and Borderline Tumours

Intramuscular Myxoma

Intramuscular myxoma is a benign, relatively rare soft tissue tumour probably derived from modified fibroblasts, which produce glucosaminoglycans forming hyaluronic acid but sparse collagen. Although the tumour is infrequently needled, it is of interest to the cytologist as it can easily be mistaken for low-grade myxoid sarcoma of various types. Intramuscular myxoma is seen in adults, most commonly between the ages of 40 and 70. Typical sites are the thigh, shoulder region and upper arm. Clinically it presents as a deep-seated, fairly circumscribed, firm to fluctuant, mobile mass. The intramuscular myxoma is a benign tumour with an extremely low recurrence rate after surgery.

Histopathology

It is a paucicellular tumour, which has an abundant myxoid, poorly vascularized stroma.

The tumour cells have characteristically slender long cytoplasmic processes and bland nuclei. Elongated cells as well as triangular cells are found. Macrophages with abundant vacuolated cytoplasm are often found among the tumour cells. The myxoma often infiltrates the surrounding striated muscle, and myxoma cells and atrophic muscle fibres are intermingled in the border zone. The FNA appearance of intramuscular myxoma has been described in individual case reports and in one series [24].

Cytological features of intramuscular myxoma (fig. 67a–c)

- Aspirates consist of droplets of colourless, stringy, glue-like fluid
- Prominent myxoid background matrix (best visualized in MGG)
- Individual, scattered vessel fragments may be seen in the background
- Dispersed cells as well as small cellular aggregates or clusters
- Tumour cells have elongated ovoid or rounded uniform, bland nuclei and long slender cytoplasmic processes
- Scattered large rounded, polyhedral or triangular cells with abundant vacuolated cytoplasm and rounded paracentral nuclei often found, corresponding to the macrophage-like cells in histological sections
- Variable presence of large multinucleated atrophic muscle fibres ('muscle giant cells')

Differential diagnosis

- Myxoid neurilemoma
- Deep-seated nodular fasciitis
- Ganglion
- Myxoid liposarcoma
- Low-grade myxofibrosarcoma
- Low-grade fibromyxoid sarcoma
- Extraskeletal myxoid chondrosarcoma

Comment

Important cytological features typical of intramuscular myxoma are a myxoid background poor in vessels, and bland cells with long, thin cytoplasmic processes. The paucity of vessels or vessel fragments speaks against myxoid liposarcoma and myxofibrosarcoma.

The uniform cells with long cytoplasmic processes are not typical of fasciitis, neurilemoma, ganglion or myxofibrosarcoma. The vacuolated cells may resemble lipoblasts but their nuclei are not scalloped.

Ancillary diagnostic methods are of little value in the differential diagnosis.

In 1998 Nielsen et al. [116] suggested the term cellular myxoma for cases of intramuscular myxoma with areas

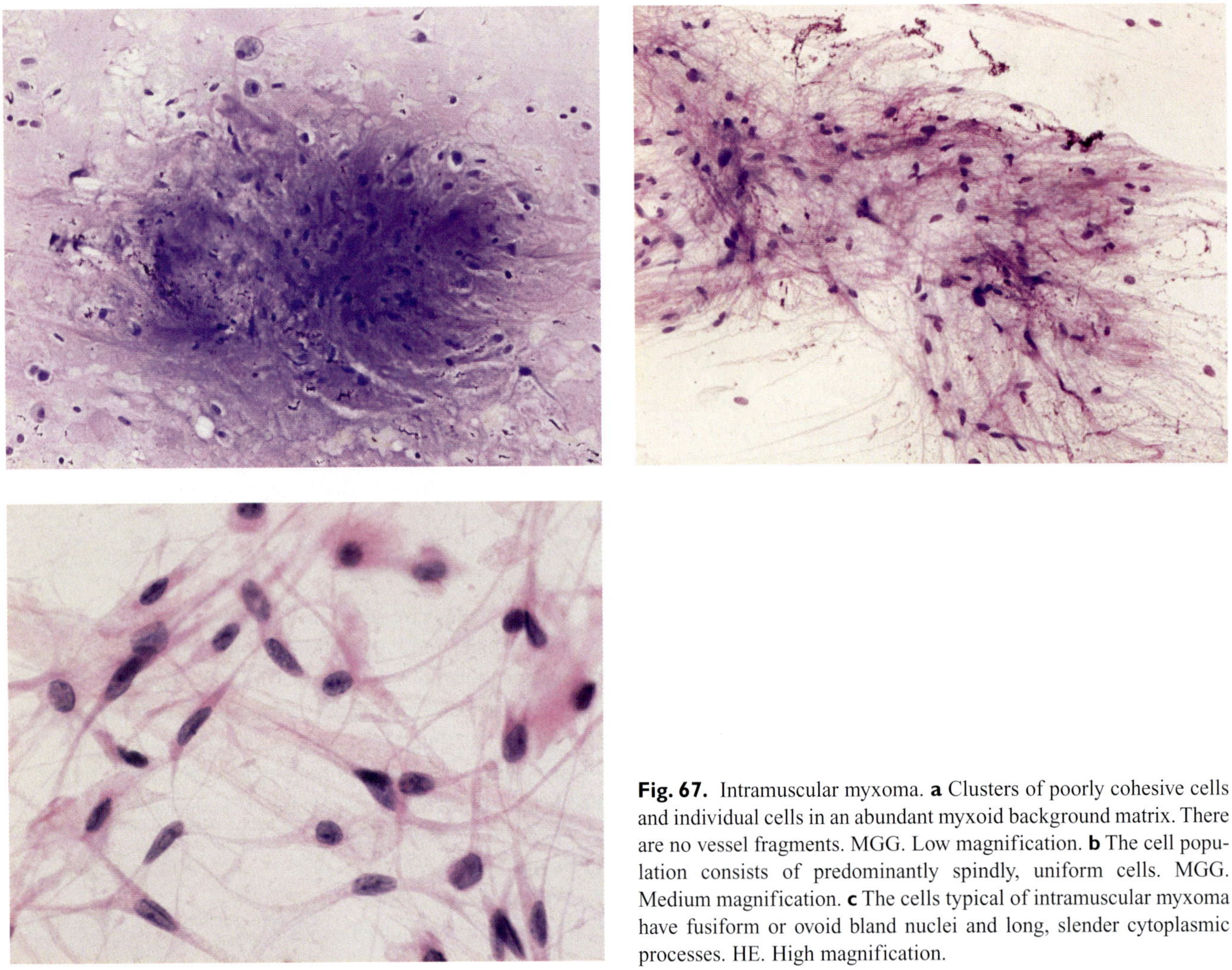

a b c

Fig. 67. Intramuscular myxoma. **a** Clusters of poorly cohesive cells and individual cells in an abundant myxoid background matrix. There are no vessel fragments. MGG. Low magnification. **b** The cell population consists of predominantly spindly, uniform cells. MGG. Medium magnification. **c** The cells typical of intramuscular myxoma have fusiform or ovoid bland nuclei and long, slender cytoplasmic processes. HE. High magnification.

of increased cellularity and hypervascularity. Another term proposed for these lesions is 'myxoid lesions with potential for recurrence' [1].

We found such cases in our FNA material (fig. 68a, b). They are difficult to distinguish from low-grade myxofibrosarcoma and low-grade fibromyxoid sarcoma due to the presence of cellular areas in the smears and of vessel fragments like those typical of myxofibrosarcoma. The FNA findings in one such lesion have been reported [117]. Another myxoma variant, which may be a diagnostic pitfall, is the juxta-articular myxoma. These tumours arise in the vicinity of the large joints and at histological examination resemble classic intramuscular myxoma. The main differential diagnosis in the cytological praxis is a ganglion.

Ossifying Fibromyxoid Tumour

This rare soft tissue tumour, first described in 1989 [118], is predominantly a tumour of adult life. It is a subcutaneous tumour, most commonly found in the extremities, although it has appeared in other sites such as the trunk and the head and neck region. The clinical behaviour is in most cases that of a benign tumour. However, rare cases have shown metastatic potential and in 1995 Kilpatrick et al. [119] reported 6 tumours, which they considered 'atypical' or malignant. The histogenesis of ossifying fibromyxoid tumour (OFMT) is debated, but schwannian differentiation has been suggested.

Histopathology

The typical OFMT is a well-circumscribed multilobated tumour with a fibrous capsule. It is composed of rather uniform rounded, ovoid or spindle-shaped cells within a stroma, variably myxoid and collagenous. The tumour cells have pale or eosinophilic cytoplasm and vesicular nuclei with small nucleoli. The rounded cells have an epithelioid appearance. In the majority of OFMT a more or less complete shell of mature, lamellar bone is present within the fibrous capsule.

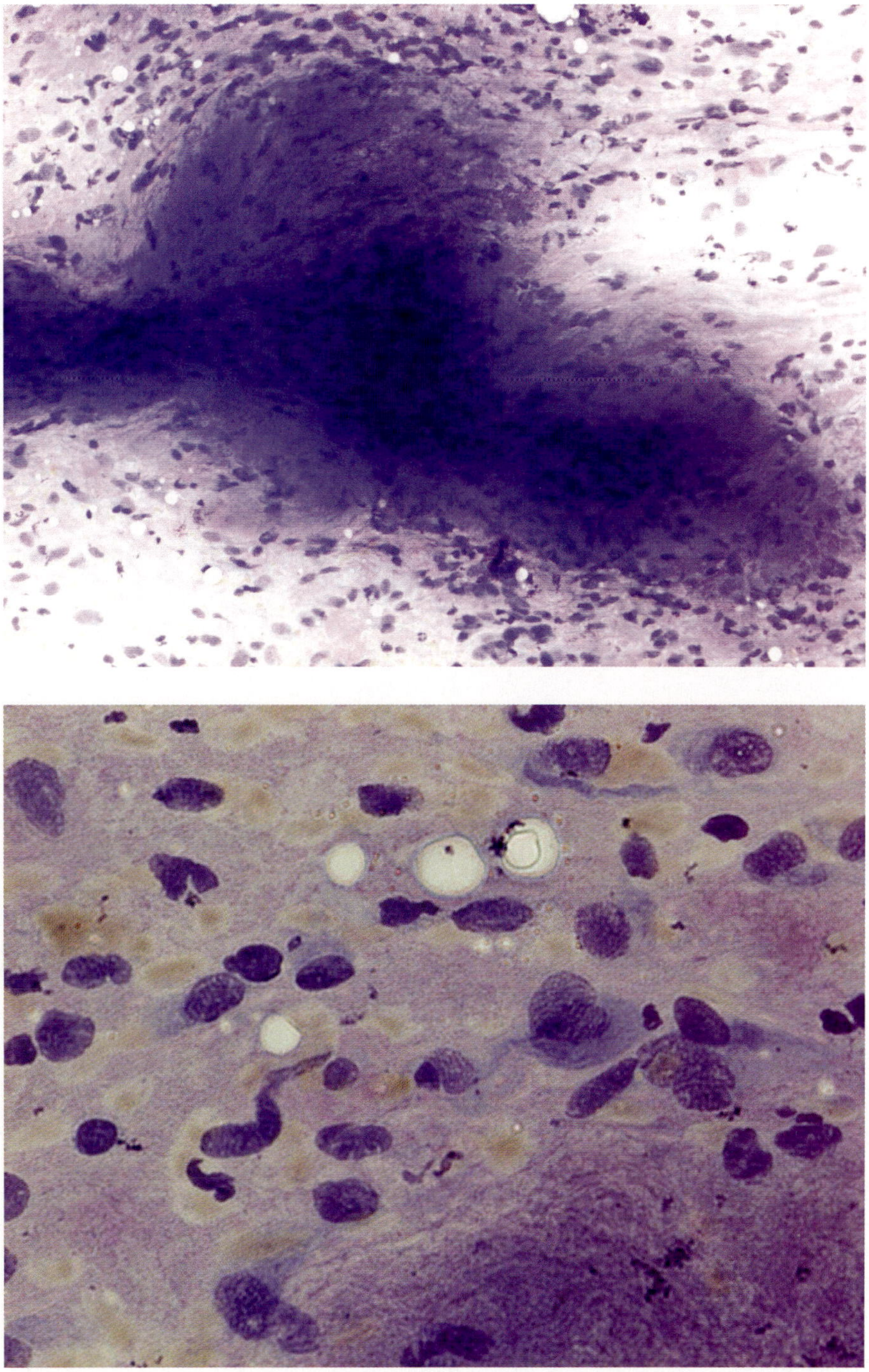

a

b

Fig. 68. Cellular myxoma ('myxoid lesion with potential for recurrence'). **a** At low magnification conventional intramuscular myxoma and cellular myxoma are remarkably alike. MGG. Low magnification. **b** In cellular myxoma, the cell population is moderately pleomorphic and includes rounded tumour cells. The distinction between cellular myxoma and low-grade malignant myxofibrosarcoma may be difficult in FNA smears. MGG. Medium magnification.

The bone component may extend into the tumour mass. Immunohistochemically, the tumour cells express S-100 protein in 60–70% of cases together with positivity for SMA in about 50%. Ultrastructurally, whorls of cytoplasmic intermediate filaments, short fragments of external laminae and interdigitating cell processes are found.

The cytology of OFMT has not yet been completely investigated. The cytological appearance has been described only in individual cases [120]. We have studied FNA smears of 1 case of OFMT.

Cytological features of OFMT (fig. 69a, b)

Variable amount of myxoid matrix and variable cellularity
Dissociated cells, cell clusters and acinar or rosette-like structures

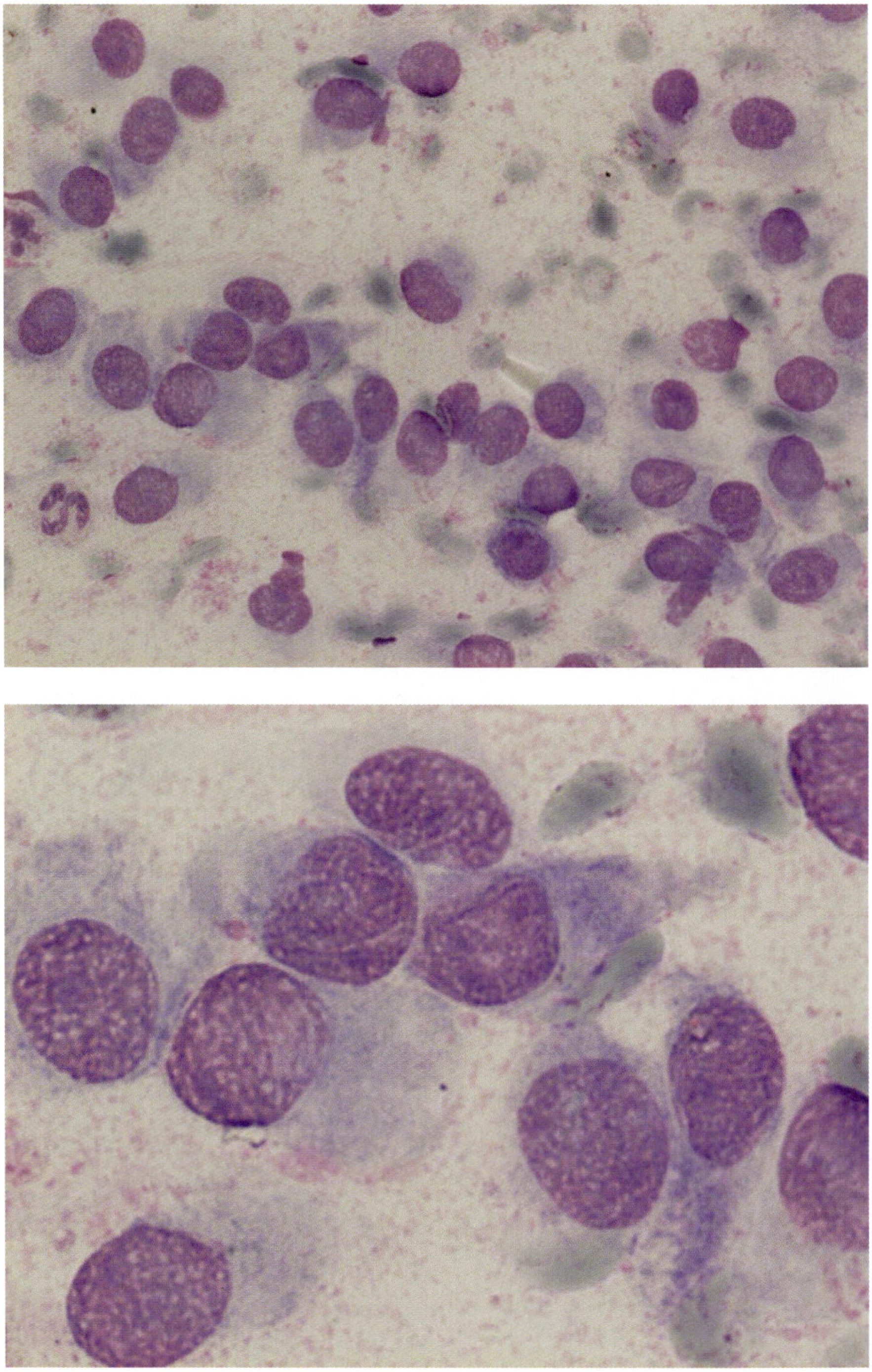

Fig. 69. OFMT. **a** Small clusters of poorly cohesive rounded cells. MGG. Low magnification. **b** The cells have rounded, at times paracentral nuclei and relatively abundant cytoplasm. MGG. High magnification.

Rounded, ovoid nuclei, at times paracentral, in a rather abundant cytoplasm

Mild nuclear pleomorphism

Differential diagnosis

The differential diagnosis includes tumours with a fibromyxoid stroma and epithelioid-like cells

Epithelioid nerve sheath tumours

Chondroid syringoma, mixed tumour of soft tissue

Extraskeletal myxoid chondrosarcoma

Epithelioid smooth muscle tumours

Thyroid neoplasms (head and neck tumours)

Comment

It is probably very difficult or impossible to obtain sufficient material for evaluation from an OFMT with a more or less complete shell of lamellar bone. Double positivity for

S-100 protein and SMA is of diagnostic help and together with negative staining for cytokeratins, desmin and caldesmon should exclude mixed tumour and smooth muscle tumour.

EM examination is probably the best method to exclude extraskeletal myxoid chondrosarcoma with regard to the paracentral whorls of intermediate filaments.

Mixed Tumour and Myoepithelioma of Soft Tissue

The occurrence of mixed tumour/myoepithelioma in soft tissue was suggested in 1997 [121]. These tumours were found mainly in the extremities of middle-aged adults, subcutaneously as well as in the deep soft tissue.

Histopathology

The tumours have the same microscopic features as pleomorphic adenoma of salivary glands or chondroid syringoma. They have a well-defined epitheial component and stain positively for cytokeratins, EMA (variably) and S-100 protein. Staining for SMA and GFAP has been recorded in some cases.

Two cases have been registered in our files.

Cytological features of mixed tumour of soft tissues (fig. 70a, b)

- Abundant myxoid background
- Tumour cells in rows, clusters or groups; glandular arrangement of cells rare
- Tumour cells variably spindle-shaped or rounded epithelioid-like

Differential diagnosis

- Chondroid syringoma
- OFMT
- Extraskeletal myxoid chondrosarcoma
- Parachordoma

Comment

The cytological features of chondroid syringoma and mixed tumour of soft tissue are remarkably alike. Cytokeratin and S-100 positivity does not help in the differential diagnosis against parachordoma. When cytokeratin is expressed together with SMA and/or GFAP, however, IC is of diagnostic help versus extraskeletal myxoid chondrosarcoma (EMC), OFMT and parachordoma.

Parachordoma

Parachordoma is a very rare benign soft tissue neoplasm of uncertain origin. It was first described in 1951. The largest series reported appeared in 1997 [122]. The reason to include this infrequent tumour is that in cytological practice parachordoma is an important differential diagnosis to extraskeletal myxoid chondrosarcoma and mixed tumour of soft tissue.

Parachordoma is a tumour of adult life; most are situated in the deep soft tissues of the extremities. The tumour has a potential for local recurrence.

Histopathology

Parachordomas are composed of nests, cords, chains and acinar-like structures of tumour cells embedded in a variably myxoid or hyaline matrix. The tumour cells are predominantly rounded, epithelioid, with insignificant atypia, but foci of spindle-shaped cells or vacuolated physaliferous-like cells are often found. The immunohistochemical profile has been described in 4 cases [122]. Parachordomas express vimentin, S-100 protein and high- molecular-weight cytokeratins. The tumour cells show primitive cell junctions and microvillous projections at electron-microscopic examination. Few cases have been studied by cytogenetic methods; specific aberrations have not been found.

It has been debated whether parachordoma is a peripheral chordoma or a variant of mixed tumour/myoepithelioma of soft tissue. However, based on the different immunophenotypes between parachordoma and chordoma, especially with regard to the cytokeratins [123] and no definitive support for myoepithelial or epithelial differentiation, parachordoma is considered to be a specific entity.

One case of primary parachordoma and one of a local recurrence are registered in our files.

Cytological features of parachordoma (fig. 71a, b)

- Abundant myxoid background
- Tumour cells both dispersed and arranged in groups, cords and runs
- Rounded, polygonal and elongated cells with fairly abundant cytoplasm; some cells have a vacuolated cytoplasm
- Rounded and ovoid bland nuclei, eccentric nuclei in vacuolated cells
- Moderate cellular pleomorphism

Differential diagnosis

- EMC
- Mixed tumour/myoepithelioma of soft tissue
- Low-grade myxofibrosarcoma
- Low-grade fibromyxoid sarcoma

Comment

The most important differential diagnoses are EMC and mixed tumour of soft tissue.

IC is of help in the differential diagnosis. In parachordoma the double positivity for cytokeratins and S-100 protein is typical. EMC very rarely marks for cytokeratins and only in 30–40% of cases for S-100 protein. Although

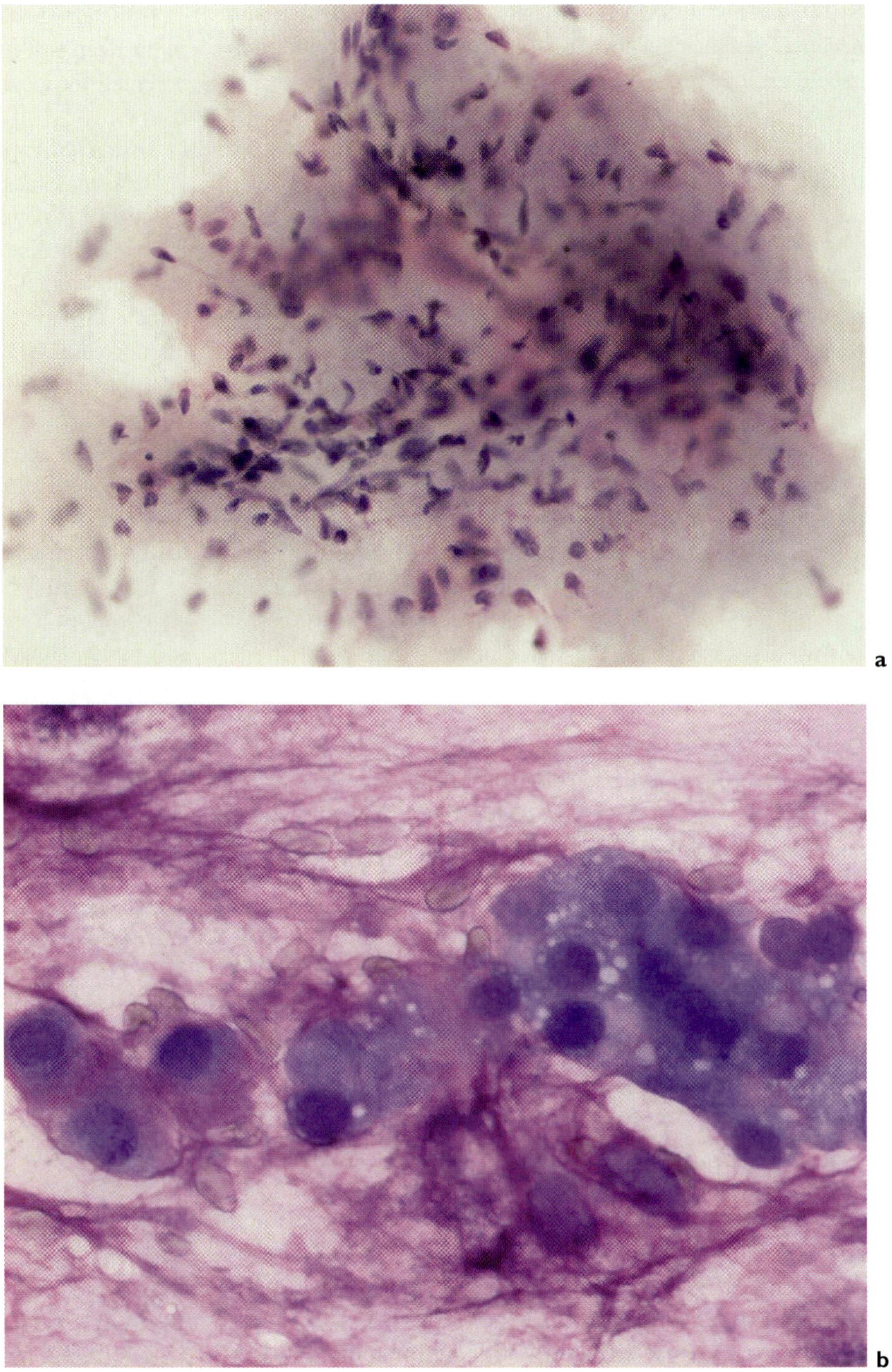

Fig. 70. Mixed tumour of soft tissue. **a** A three-dimensional tissue fragment composed of cells embedded in a myxoid matrix. HE. Low magnification. **b** The chondromyxoid matrix is evident in MGG-stained smears. The myxoid matrix and the constitutional cells in this case resemble the pleomorphic adenoma of the salivary gland. MGG. Medium magnification.

both parachordoma and mixed tumour of soft tissue stain for S-100 protein and cytokeratins, parachordoma does not express SMA or GFAP. Cytokeratin positivity also excludes myxofibrosarcomas and fibromyxoid sarcomas. Furthermore, low-grade myxofibrosarcoma and fibromyxoid sarcoma are mainly composed of spindle cells exhibiting slight atypia.

Malignant Tumours

Desmoplastic Small Round Cell Tumour

Although this relatively rare malignant neoplasm has been reported to arise in various anatomical sites such as the parotid gland, thoracic region and CNS, the overwhelming majority of cases are found in the abdominal and/or pelvic

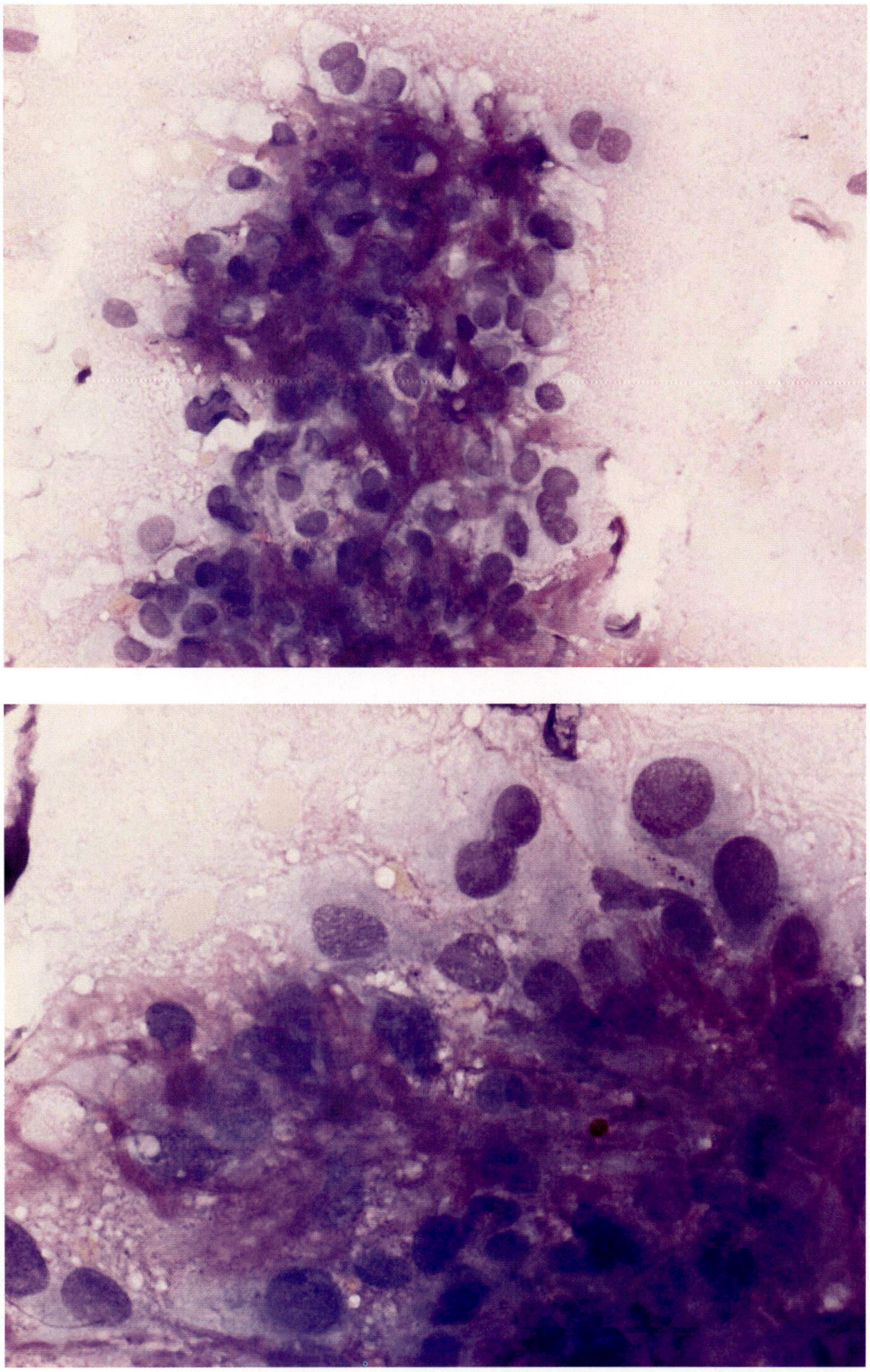

a

b

Fig. 71. Parachordoma. **a** A tight cluster of rounded and polygonal cells embedded in an abundant myxoid matrix. Many cells have an abundant, clear or vacuolated cytoplasm. MGG. Medium magnification. **b** The tumour cells are moderately pleomorphic. MGG. High magnification.

peritoneum. Young males are most often affected. Most patients are between 15 and 35 years of age.

DSRCT is a highly malignant polyphenotypic neoplasm of unknown histogenesis.

Histopathology

Nests and groups of small to medium-sized cells are seen within a fibrous, vascularized stroma. Central necrosis is not uncommon in larger nests. The tumour cells have scanty cytoplasm and rounded hyperchromatic nuclei with small nucleoli. Foci of rhabdoid tumour cells with relatively abundant cytoplasm and paranuclear inclusions may be found.

The typical immunohistochemical profile is expression of cytokeratins, EMA, desmin and NSE. The cytokeratin and desmin positivity often appears as perinuclear dots.

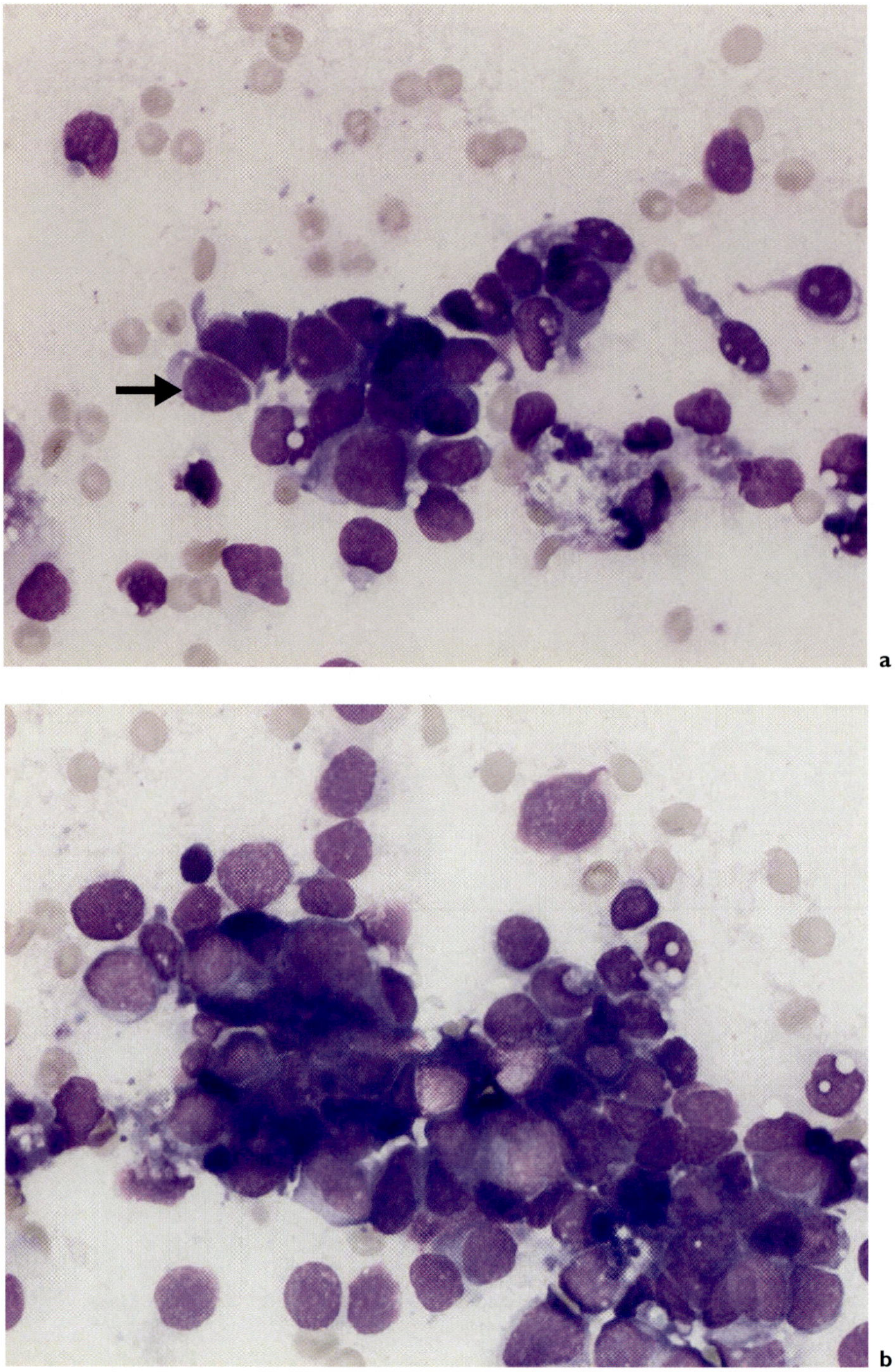

Fig. 72. Desmoplastic small round cell tumour. **a** Tumour cells in an epithelial-like arrangement. An acinus-like structure (arrow) and Indian files. MGG. High magnification. **b** The tumour cells are small to medium-sized with rounded nuclei and scant cytoplasm. The chromatin is finely granular. MGG. High magnification.

Ultrastructurally the most striking finding is perinuclear cytoplasmic whorls of filaments.

A specific cytogenetic abnormality has been reported in DSRCT, t(11;22)(p13;q12) involving the EWS gene on 22q12 and the WT1 gene on 11p13. Recently a polyclonal anti-WT1 antibody, detecting the WT1 protein, has been tested with promising diagnostic results [124].

The cytomorphology of DSRCT has been described in a series of 4 cases and in reports of individual cases [125–127].

Cytological features of DSRCT (fig. 72a, b)

Tumour cells arranged in loosely cohesive clusters or in epithelial-like groups

Small to medium-sized rounded or ovoid tumour cells with scant cytoplasm
Rounded or ovoid nuclei with finely granular chromatin and small nucleoli
Clusters of fibroblast-like stromal cells may be found

Differential diagnosis
ES/PNET
Alveolar rhabdomyosarcoma
Small cell carcinoma
Malignant mesothelioma
Non-Hodgkin's lymphoma

Comment

As the typical pattern in biopsy material (cell nests in a fibrous stroma) is difficult to appreciate in FNA smears (co-existence of small malignant cells and fibroblast-like cells in smears from an abdominal tumour may suggest the diagnosis), ancillary tests should be done before a definitive diagnosis is made.

The typical polyphenotypic profile (cytokeratin, EMA, desmin and NSE) is a valuable diagnostic adjunct. DSRCT has been reported to express CD99 in a number of cases. The WT1 antibody has not yet, to our knowledge, been tested in cytological material.

Ultrastructurally, paranuclear whorls of filaments are not found in ES/PNET, mesothelioma or lymphoma. Thick and thin filaments and Z-bands as in alveolar rhabdomyosarcoma are not seen in DSRCT.

Regarding cytogenetics and molecular genetics, the t(11;22)(p13;q12) is an important diagnostic aid in relation to carcinoma, mesothelioma, alveolar rhabdomyosarcoma and lymphoma. However, FISH of the common EWS breakpoint does not discriminate between ES/PNET and DSRCT. Although DSRCT is a rare tumour, it is always an alternative differential diagnosis when FNA smears from large intra-abdominal masses in younger males show a malignant small cell population.

Malignant Extrarenal Rhabdoid Tumour

It has been debated whether malignant extrarenal rhabdoid tumour of soft tissue exists as a specific clinicopathological entity originating from multipotential, primitive cells, or whether cells with rhabdoid morphology are part of the cell population in a number of malignant tumours with a proven line of differentiation. Examples are various carcinomas, malignant melanoma, rhabdomyosarcoma, leiomyosarcoma, synovial sarcoma and desmoplastic small round cell tumour. The current opinion, however, is that extrarenal rhabdoid tumour of soft tissue should be regarded as a specific entity in cases with a predominant rhabdoid morphology and no specific line of differentiation.

Histopathology

Rhabdoid morphology includes large polygonal cells with paracentral nuclei, vesicular chromatin, large nucleoli and acidophilic and PAS-positive hyaline inclusions in an abundant cytoplasm.

Ultrastructurally the inclusions correspond to paranuclear masses composed of whorls of intermediate filaments. The immunophenotype is, to some extent, similar to that of DSRCT. Extrarenal rhabdoid tumours express cytokeratins, vimentin and neuroectodermal antibodies such as NSE, but not desmin.

A few reports on the cytological features of malignant extrarenal rhabdoid tumour in FNA have been published [128, 129]. Our own experience corresponds with the cases reported.

Cytological features of extrarenal rhabdoid tumour (fig. 73a, b)
Cell clusters and dispersed cells
Mainly medium-sized to large rounded, triangular or polygonal cells with abundant cytoplasm
Large rounded or bean-shaped nuclei with prominent nucleoli
Paranuclear cytoplasmic globular inclusions, grey-blue in MGG, faintly acidophilic in HE

Differential diagnosis
Rhabdomyosarcoma
Epithelioid sarcoma
Malignant melanoma
Poorly differentiated synovial sarcoma
Undifferentiated large cell carcinoma

Comment

It is not difficult to diagnose extrarenal rhabdoid tumour as a high-grade malignant neoplasm in FNA smears. However, for a specific diagnosis to be made, other malignancies, which may be partly composed of tumour cells with rhabdoid morphology, have to be excluded.

Alveolar Soft Part Sarcoma

This uncommon sarcoma, first described in 1952, is estimated to account for up to 1% of soft tissue sarcomas. In spite of its rarity it is of interest as an alternative differential diagnosis to more frequent tumours such as granular cell tumour and metastasis of renal carcinoma.

Alveolar soft part sarcoma is mainly found in adolescents and young adults. In children the favoured site is the head

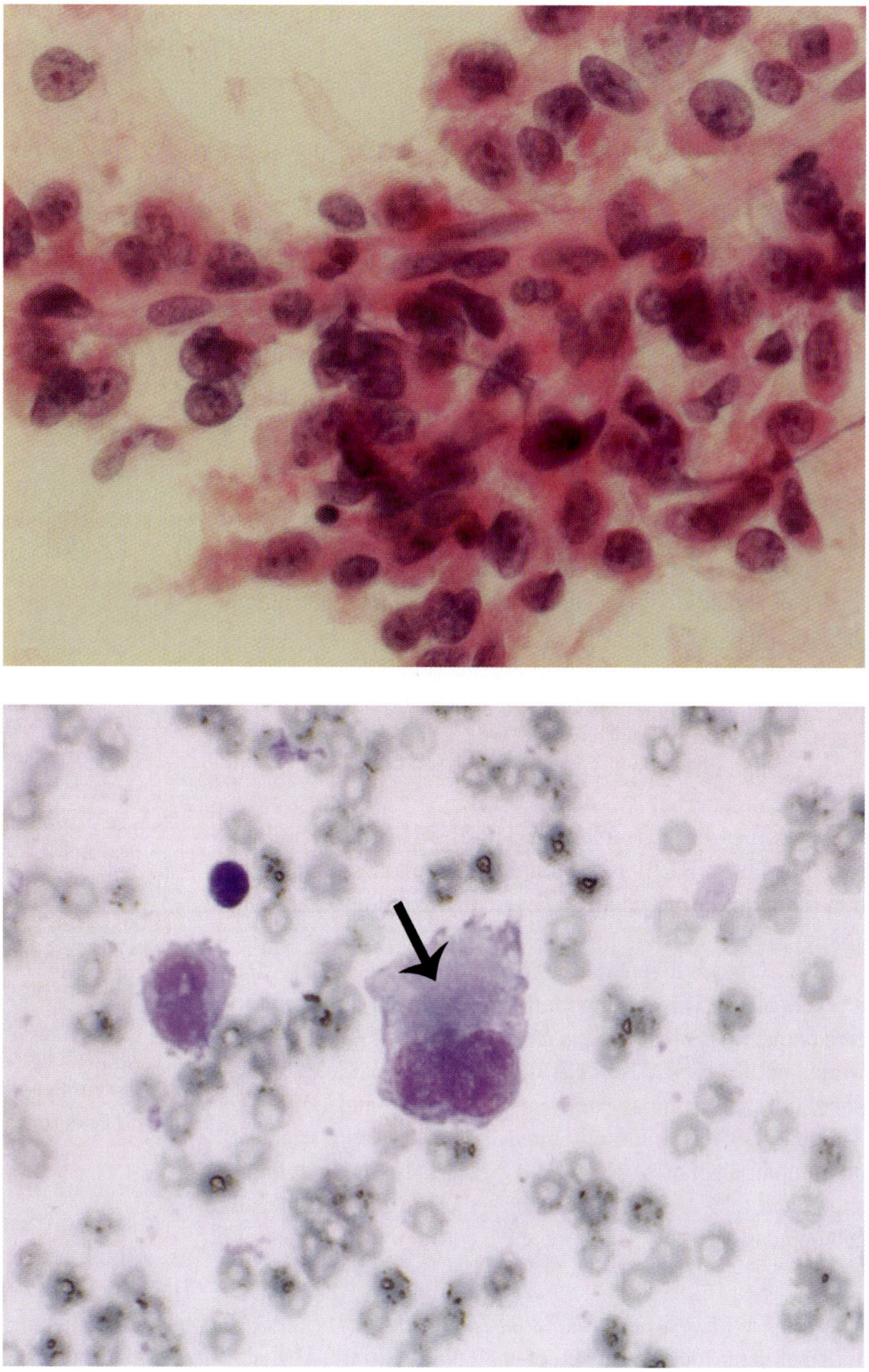

a

b

Fig. 73. Malignant extrarenal rhabdoid tumour. **a** A tight cluster of rounded or polygonal cells with relatively abundant cytoplasm and rounded nuclei. HE. Medium magnification. **b** Individual cells are triangular with eccentric nuclei and abundant cytoplasm. There is an indistinct grey-blue cytoplasmic globular inclusion (arrow). MGG, oil.

and neck region, including orbit and tongue, and in adults the most frequent site is the legs and buttocks.

Histopathology

Alveolar soft part sarcoma is characteristically lobulated and composed of groups or sheets of cells divided by fibrous septa. An organoid pseudoalveolar pattern is common. The stroma is rich in sinusoidal-like vascular channels. Individual tumour cells are typically large, rounded or polygonal with abundant cytoplasm. Nuclei are rounded with prominent nucleoli. The cytoplasm is mostly granular and in the majority of tumours contains characteristic rod-shaped or rhomboid crystals, which are PAS-positive.

Reported results of immunohistochemical staining are contradictonary. However, in most series, a variable positivity for vimentin, muscle-specific actin, SMA and desmin has been recorded while cytokeratins, EMA and S-100 protein are negative. Electron-microscopic findings are similar in the different cases. Numerous mitochondria, glycogen deposits, a well-developed Golgi apparatus and characteristic crystals with a lattice-like pattern have been described. A specific diagnostic cytogenetic aberration has not been found.

The histogenesis of alveolar soft tissue sarcoma is not clear. Skeletal muscle differentiation is the most favoured hypothesis. The cytological features of alveolar soft part sarcoma have been investigated in a few publications [50, 51]. The cytopathology of the 2 cases in our files is similar to published reports.

Cytological features of alveolar soft part sarcoma (fig. 74a, b)

- Haemorrhagic samples
- Cells in clusters and dispersed
- Stripped nuclei and a cytoplasmic background substance are common
- Intact cells are epithelioid, large, rounded or polyhedral
- The cytoplasm is often granular
- Binucleated and multinucleated cells are not uncommon
- Rounded nuclei with prominent central nucleoli
- The rod-shaped crystals are rarely identified

Differential diagnosis

- Renal cell carcinoma
- Paraganglioma
- Granular cell tumour
- Rhabdomyoma

Comment

In our opinion, granular cell tumour is the most important differential diagnosis. Both tumours commonly exhibit stripped nuclei, which are rounded with a central prominent nucleolus. In both tumours intact cells have granular cytoplasm.

Granular cell tumours are typically S-100 protein-positive and desmin- and SMA-negative.

Ultrastructurally granular cell tumours are characterized by large autophagic granules.

Epithelioid Sarcoma

Epithelioid sarcoma is a distinctive clinicopathological entity occurring mainly in the extremities and especially in the distal parts, in adolescents and young adults. Epithelioid sarcoma is rarely found in the trunk or in the head and neck. It is located in the subcutis or in the deeper soft tissues. Subcutaneous tumours typically present as slow-growing, firm nodules. The nodules often became ulcerated. Deep-seated lesions involve tendons, tendon sheaths and fasciae in an infiltrating manner.

Histopathology

There is a nodular arrangement of tumour cells, often with central necrosis. Aggregates of lymphocytes, plasma cells and histiocytes surround the tumour noduli. The stroma is variably collagenous and hyalinized. The sarcoma cells are pleomorphic, ranging from large rounded or polyhedral epithelioid forms to plump spindle-shaped cells. The cytoplasm is eosinophilic (mainly the epithelioid cells) or may contain intracytoplasmic lipid droplets. The nuclei are rounded, ovoid or spindly with more or less prominent nucleoli.

A 'proximal' type of epithelioid sarcoma has been described; in this variety cells with rhabdoid features dominate [130].

The tumour cells stain for low- and high-molecular-weight cytokeratins, EMA and vimentin in the majority of cases. The immunoreactivity may be focal in a specific tumour and the degree of positivity varies between different tumours. About 70% stain for CD34 while S-100 protein, CD31 and factor VIII are negative. The most striking ultrastructural finding is paranuclear masses or whorls of intermediate filaments. Desmosome-like junctions may be seen.

Various abnormalities have been described in the limited number of tumours that have been cytogenetically investigated, but no specific aberration of diagnostic significance.

Due to the subcutaneous location, the nodularity, central ulceration and the inflammatory cell infiltrate one important differential diagnosis is a benign granulomatous lesion. Other differential diagnoses include epithelioid MPNST, malignant melanoma, epithelioid angiosarcoma and squamous cell carcinoma.

There is at present no consensus as regards the origin of epithelioid sarcoma. Fibroblastic, histiocytic, synovial and myofibroblastic origins have ben proposed. The cytological features of epithelioid sarcoma have been investigated in a series of 9 cases and in case reports [55, 56].

Cytological features of epithelioid sarcoma (fig. 75a–c)

- Variable numbers of sarcoma cells
- Both cellular clusters and dispersed cells seen in abundant smears
- Necrosis

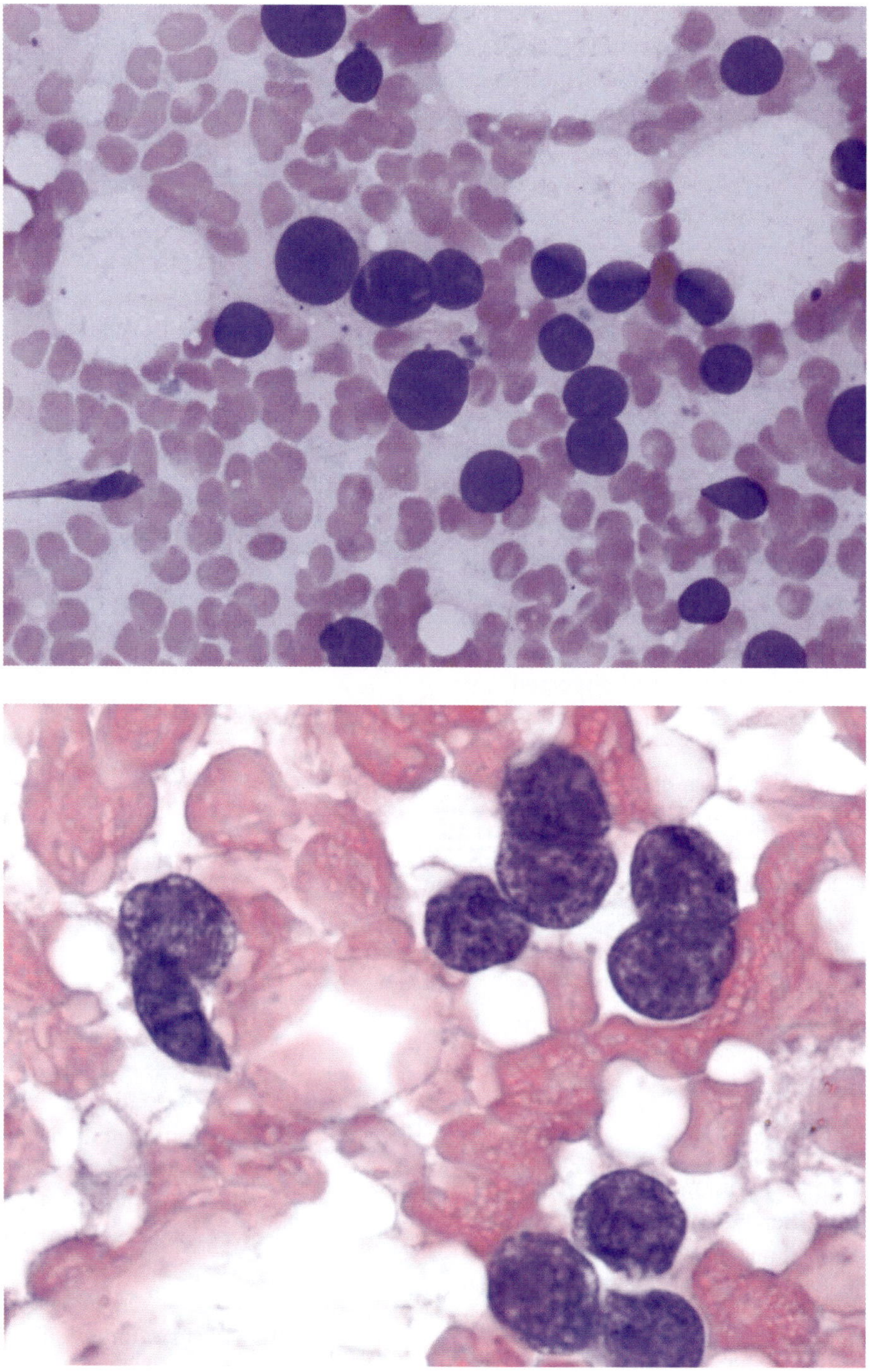

Fig. 74. Alveolar soft part sarcoma. **a** Numerous stripped nuclei are a common feature in FNA smears. Note the faintly stained cytoplasmic background substance. MGG. Medium magnification. **b** The nuclei have prominent nucleoli. HE. High magnification.

Medium-sized to large rounded, polygonal or spindle-shaped tumour cells with variable amount of fragile cytoplasm
Rounded ovoid or fusiform nuclei with large nucleoli
Admixture of variable numbers of lymphocytes, plasma cells and histiocytes

Differential diagnosis

Benign granulomatous lesions
Malignant melanoma
Sarcomas with epithelioid-like tumour cells
Squamous cell carcinoma

Comment

The most striking phenomenon recorded in the few cases in our files was the difficulty to aspirate a

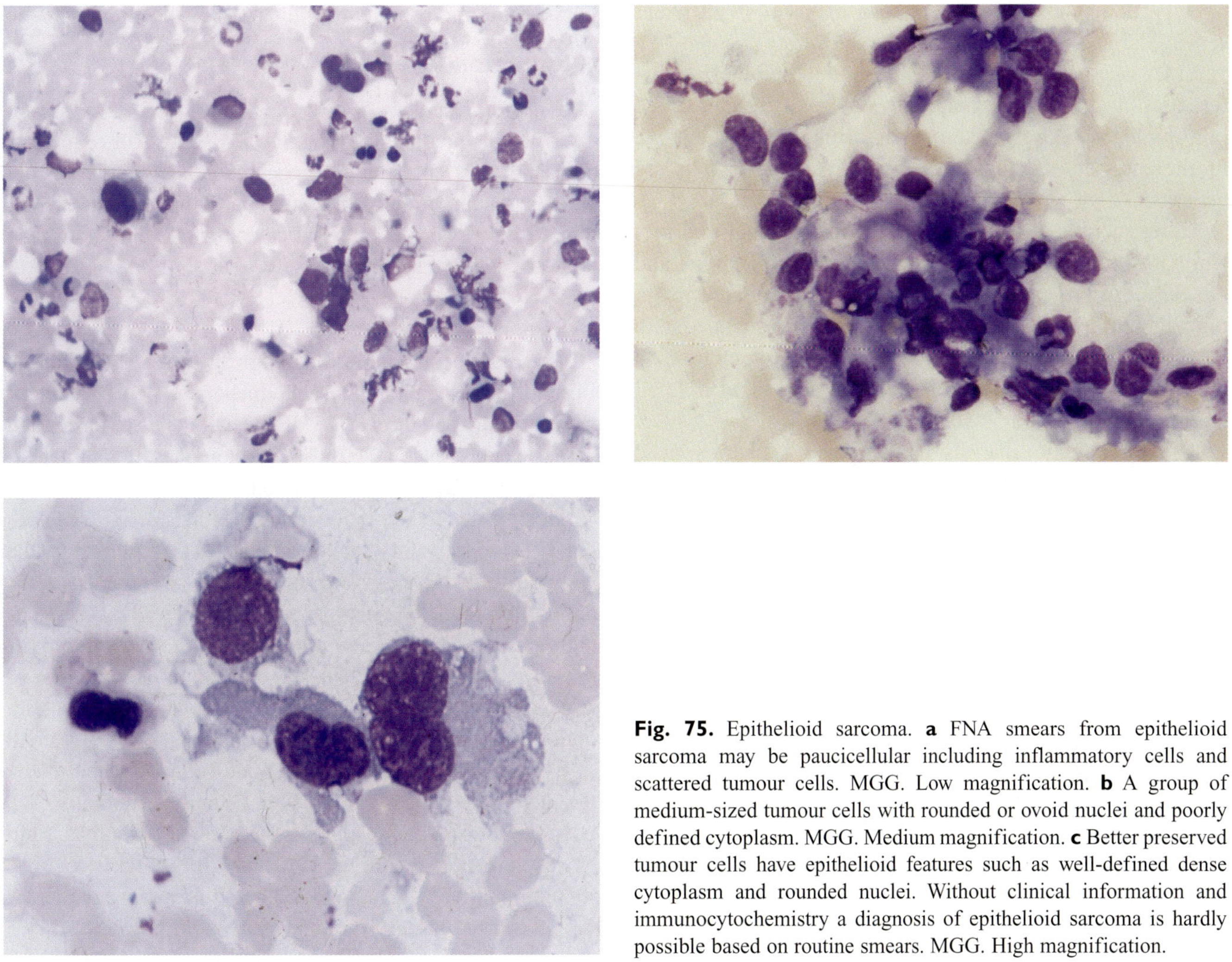

a b c

Fig. 75. Epithelioid sarcoma. **a** FNA smears from epithelioid sarcoma may be paucicellular including inflammatory cells and scattered tumour cells. MGG. Low magnification. **b** A group of medium-sized tumour cells with rounded or ovoid nuclei and poorly defined cytoplasm. MGG. Medium magnification. **c** Better preserved tumour cells have epithelioid features such as well-defined dense cytoplasm and rounded nuclei. Without clinical information and immunocytochemistry a diagnosis of epithelioid sarcoma is hardly possible based on routine smears. MGG. High magnification.

sufficiently cellular yield for thorough examination. The most important pitfall is to mistake an epithelioid sarcoma for a benign inflammatory (granulomatous) lesion. In scanty smears the inflammatory cells may dominate and the few tumour cells may be mistaken for epithelioid histiocytes. If smears are abundant, a diagnosis of malignancy is the rule.

Extraskeletal Myxoid Chondrosarcoma

EMC is a rare distinct entity, estimated to represent less than 3% of soft tissue saromas. It is a sarcoma mainly of middle-aged adults but sporadic cases occur in children. Typical sites are extremities (especially proximal parts), limb girdles and trunk. The majority of tumours are deep-seated. EMC is considered to be of chondroblastic origin, but it has recently been proposed that a proportion of EMC have neuroendocrine features [131].

Histopathology

Characteristically, EMC is a multilobular well-circumscribed tumour with a pushing tumour margin. The cells are arranged in branchingx strands, rings or ball-like clusters embedded in an abundant myxoid matrix. In classic EMC, cells are rounded or elongated with a moderate amount of cytoplasm and rounded or ovoid nuclei. The nuclei have finely dispersed chromatin and small nucleoli. There are also spindle-shaped cells with elongated nuclei.

Chondroblastoma-like bean-shaped or indented nuclei may also be present.

A subset of EMC is characterized by hypercellularity, scant myxoid stroma and tumour cells which are either small with rounded nuclei and scant cytoplasm or large with rhabdoid-like morphology. EMC has no distinct immunohistochemical profile. S-100 protein-positive tumour cells have been demonstrated in 20–75% of cases in different series. Staining is often focal.

EMA is positive in up to 25% and neuroendocrine differentiation (NSE and synaptophysin) has been described in a number of cases. Staining for cytokeratin is negative in the majority of tumours and SMA and desmin are negative.

Ultrastructurally, cells of classic EMC are enclosed in a fibrillary matrix. The cytoplasm has short projections and typically exhibits prominent Golgi zones and dilated rough reticulum, often filled with granular material associated with numerous mitochondria. Neuroendocrine differentiation in the form of neurosecretory granulae is present in a small number of cases.

The cytogenetic analysis has revealed a characteristic translocation t(9;22)(q22;q12). This translocation involves the EWS gene at 22q12 and the CHN gene at 9q22. The cytological features of EMC have been described in a small series and in case reports [132–134].

The published cases are all examples of classic EMC. One case in our files showed signs of neuroendocrine differentiation [134].

Cytological features of EMC (fig. 76a–d)

- Abundant myxoid background
- Variable arrangement of tumour cells: clusters, branching strands, cell balls and dispersed cells
- Often a central core of branching capillaries in the clusters
- Cells are variably rounded, elongated and fusiform
- Nuclei are rounded, ovoid or thin, spindle-shaped
- Chondroblastoma-like nuclei with nuclear folds or indentations (coffee bean nuclei) are often observed

Differential diagnosis

- Classic EMC
  - Intramuscular myxoma
  - Mixed tumour of soft tissue
  - Myxoid liposarcoma
  - Low-grade myxofibrosarcoma
  - Low-grade fibromyxoid sarcoma
  - Parachordoma
- Solid, hypercellular EMC
  - ES/PNET
  - Poorly differentiated synovial sarcoma

Comment

IC is of limited value as S-100 protein positivity is present in less than 50% of tumours. A broad panel of antibodies is, however, helpful to exclude epithelial, neuroectodermal and schwannian differentiation.

Electron-microscopic examination is a useful diagnostic cytological examination [68].

Synovial Sarcoma

Synovial sarcoma accounts for 5–10% of soft tissue sarcomas. It can occur at any age including childhood, but is most common in young and middle-aged adults. The majority arises in the extremities and trunk, and more than 90% are deep-seated.

Histopathology

There are four main histological types: monophasic fibrous, biphasic, monophasic epithelial and poorly differentiated (focally or entirely) [135]. The monophasic fibrous and biphasic subtypes are the most common ones, the monophasic epithelial subtype is uncommon.

Most of the cells are either spindle-shaped, uniform with scanty cytoplasm and ovoid bland nuclei or fibrosarcoma-like with fusiform nuclei. Three morphological variants of the poorly differentiated subtype have been described. One has high-grade malignant spindle cells with hyperchromatic nuclei and enlarged nucleoli. Another type is composed of large epithelioid cells, at times with rhabdoid features, with rounded nuclei and prominent nucleoli. Finally there is a small cell variant with scant cytoplasm and rounded bland nuclei resembling the cells of the ES/PNET family of tumours.

Immunohistochemically, most synovial sarcomas stain positively for cytokeratins (CK7 and CK19) and EMA. The staining may be focal, and both cytokeratins and EMA should be used as some tumours stain only for EMA and vice versa. More than half are positive for CD99 and Bcl-2 protein positivity has been reported in 70–90% of tumours. Up to a third stain for S-100 protein.

Important ultrastructural features include junctions or desmosome-like structures, and small pseudoglandular spaces bordered by short microvilli.

The majority of synovial sarcomas, including poorly differentiated tumours, share a distinct chromosomal aberration, t(X;18)(p11;q11.2). The translocation involves the SYT gene on chromosome 18 and the SSX gene family on the X chromosome. There are two major gene fusions, SYT/SSX1 and SYT/SSX2. According to two reported series of tumours, the SYT/SSX2 variant is biologically more aggressive than the SYT/SSX1 variant [136, 137].

The cytological features of synovial sarcoma have been evaluated in some series of tumours and in numerous case reports. Above all the monophasic fibrous and biphasic variants have been investigated [35–38]. Individual case reports describing the cytological features of poorly differentiated synovial sarcoma have been published [138]. Recently we had the opportunity to study FNA smears from 37 primary synovial sarcomas [139], including 6 cases of poorly differentiated tumours. The cytomorphology of our cases essentially agreed with reported series.

Cytological features of monophasic and biphasic synovial sarcoma (fig. 77a–g)

Cellular yield

Both dispersed cells and branching tumour tissue fragments of tightly packed cells

A central core of branching capillaries often present in the tumour fragments (haemangiopericytoma-like pattern)

Many stripped nuclei

Small acinar-like structures in biphasic tumours

Relatively uniform rounded or ovoid medium-sized cells with rounded, ovoid or elongated nuclei

Bland nuclear chromatin and inconspicuous nucleoli

Mitotic figures (including atypical) common in tumour fragments

Variable admixture of mast cells

Rarely myxoid background substance

Cytological features of synovial sarcoma with poorly differentiated morphology

A similar pattern of dispersed cells and tumour tissue fragments as in monophasic and biphasic tumours

Small rounded cells with scanty cytoplasm and rounded bland nuclei

Spindle-shaped cells with fusiform atypical, hyperchromatic nuclei

Large cells with rounded nuclei, prominent nucleoli and abundant cytoplasm, occasionally with rhabdoid features (eccentric nucleus, cytoplasmic inclusion)

Differential diagnosis

Solitary fibrous tumour

Malignant haemangiopericytoma

Fibrosarcoma

MPNST

Poorly differentiated variant

ES/PNET family of tumours

Alveolar rhabdomyosarcoma

Malignant rhabdoid tumour

Tumours with poor cell yield

Desmoid fibromatosis

Comment

Typical cellular smears of the synovial sarcoma are readily recognized as sarcoma. If the yield is highly cellular with a typical pattern of cellular tissue fragments and dispersed cells, the main differential diagnosis is between haemangiopericytoma, solitary fibrous tumour, and monophasic synovial sarcoma. If the smears are paucicellular showing only small runs or clusters of spindle cells, it is difficult to distinguish the tumour from other spindle cell neoplasms such as desmoid fibromatosis.

IC may not be diagnostically helpful in view of the occasionally very focal staining for cytokeratins and EMA. FISH and/or RT-PCR are the most effective adjuncts in the diagnosis of the poorly differentiated type. Furthermore, with RT-PCR it is possible to diagnose the type of gene fusion [65].

Clear Cell Sarcoma

Clear cell sarcoma, also called malignant melanoma of soft parts, is a malignant soft tissue tumour showing melanocytic differentiation. It occurs most frequently in young adults, but has been reported in children and in the elderly. The most frequent sites are the lower extremities (foot, knee and thigh) followed by the hand and wrist region. It is seldom reported in the trunk or in the head and neck. Clear cell sarcoma is usually a deep-seated lesion related to tendons and fasciae.

Histopathology

Clear cell sarcoma is usually a lobulated tumour, which has a typical histological pattern. The sarcoma cells are usually arranged in groups, nests or elongated packages surrounded by bands of fibrous tissue. They are medium-sized or large cells, variably rounded, polygonal or spindly with rounded, ovoid or fusiform nuclei. There is generally a moderate degree of nuclear pleomorphism, the cytoplasm is more often eosinophilic than clear, and the nucleoli are large and prominent. Multinucleated tumour giant cells with a wreath-like arrangement of nuclei are present in a number of tumours. Cytoplasmic melanin pigment is occasionally seen in routine stains and more than half of the tumours stain positively for melanin stains.

Immunohistochemically, the majority of clear cell sarcomas stain positively for S-100 and HMB45. Positivity for Melan A is also found. EM examination reveals premelanosomes and melanosomes in many tumour cells. About three fourths of clear cell sarcomas display a chromosomal aberration t(12;22)(q13–14;q12–13) involving the *ATF1* gene on chromosome 12 and the *EWS* gene on chromosome 22.

The cytology of clear cell sarcoma in FNA samples has been recorded in a small series of cases [52]. The cytology seen in the cases in our files agrees with published descriptions.

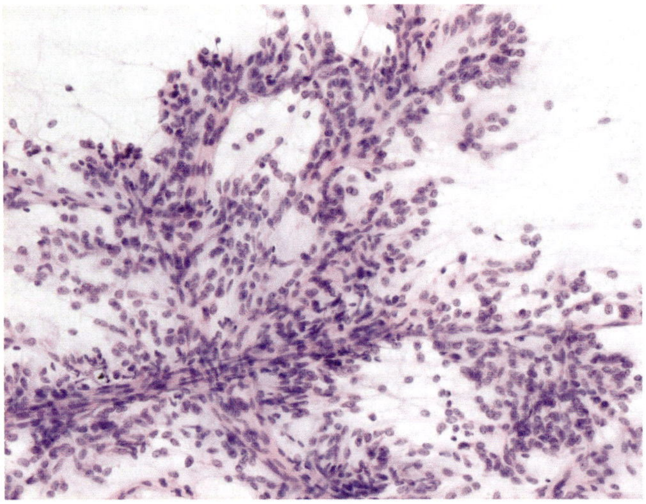

76a

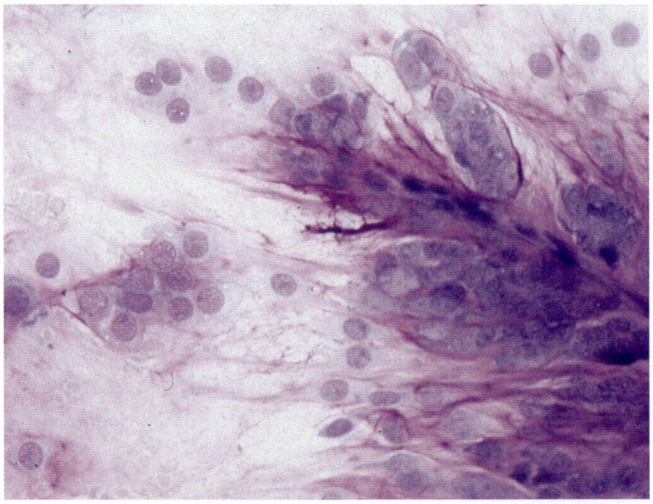

76b

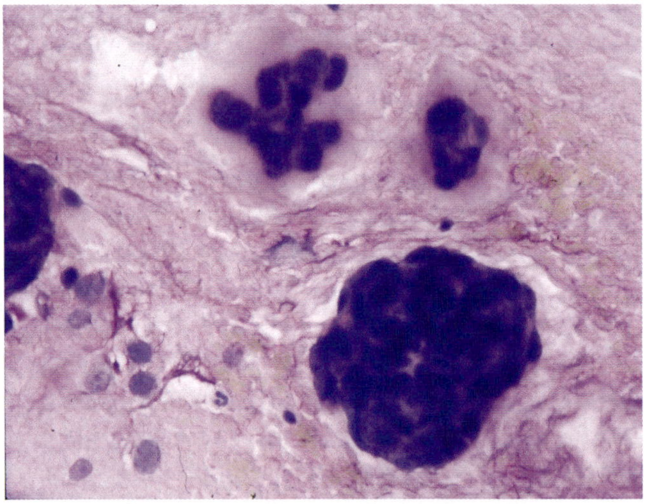

76c

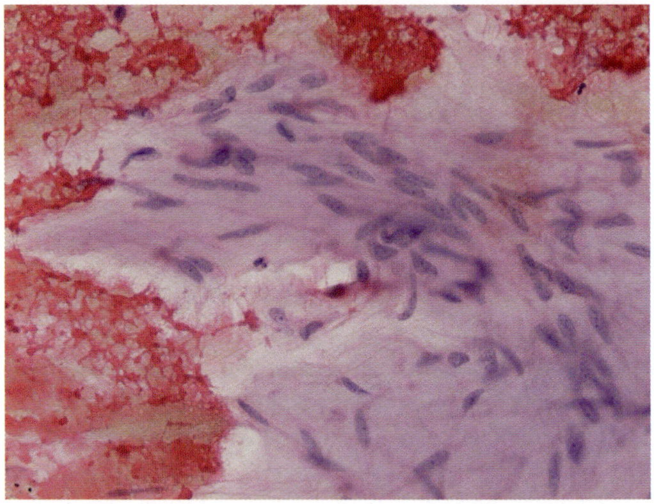

76d

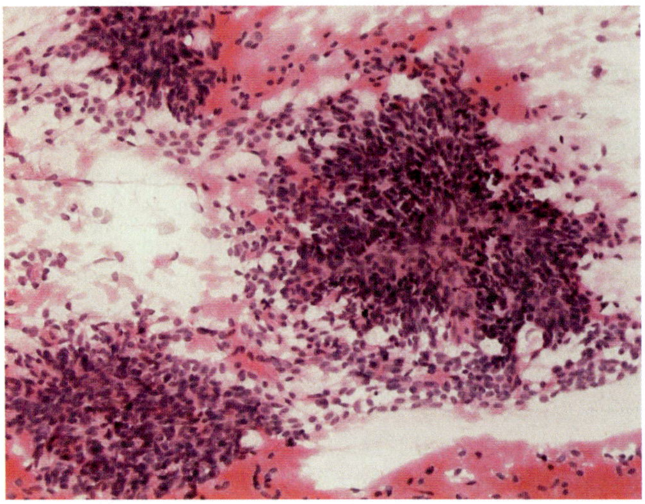

77a

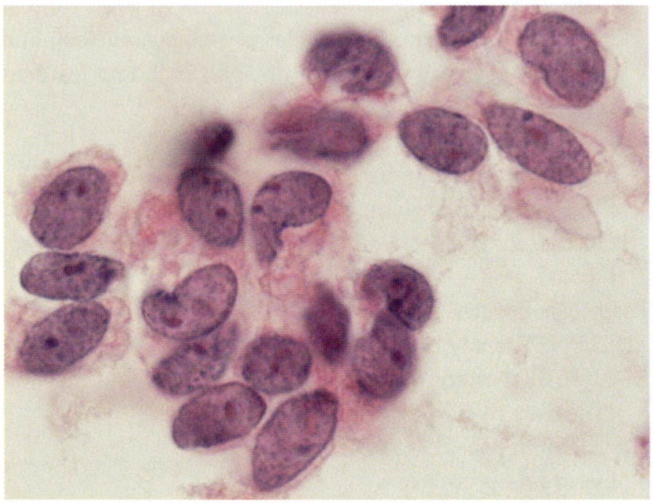

77b

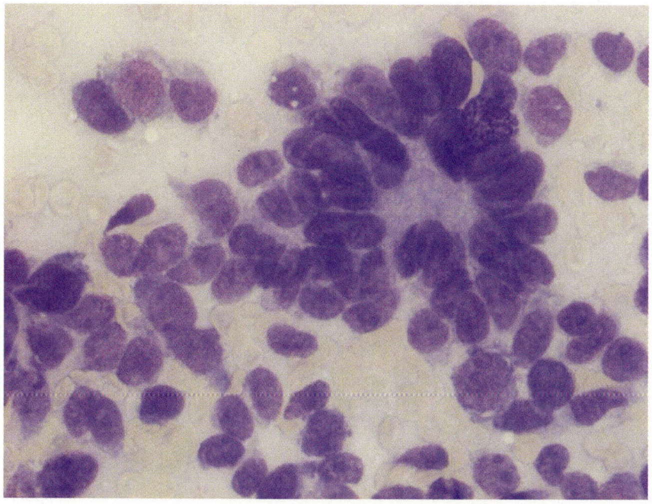
77c

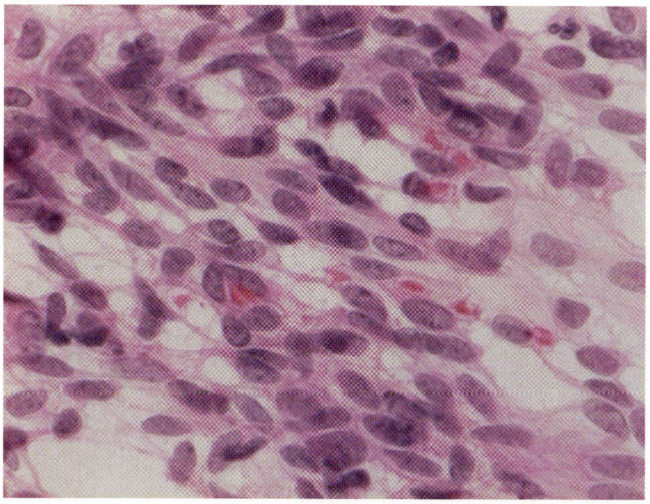
77d

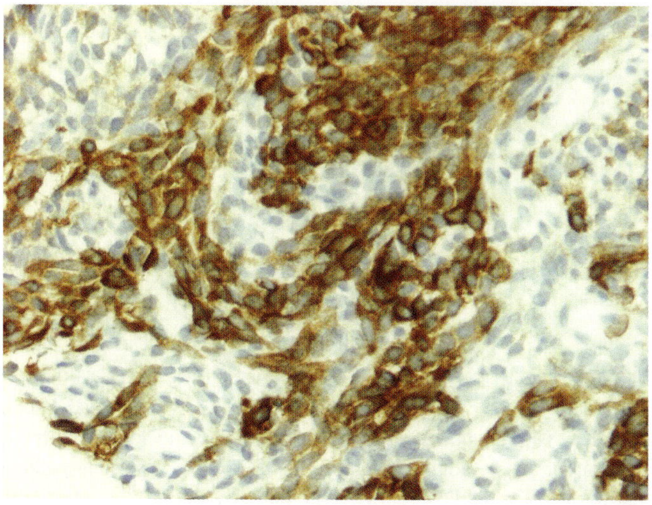
77e

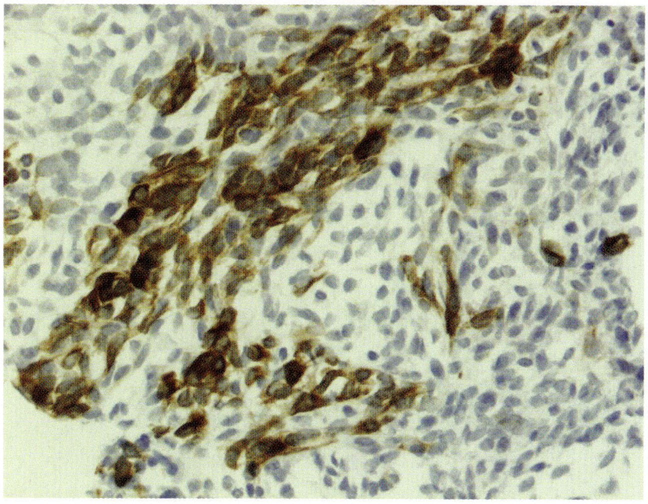
77f

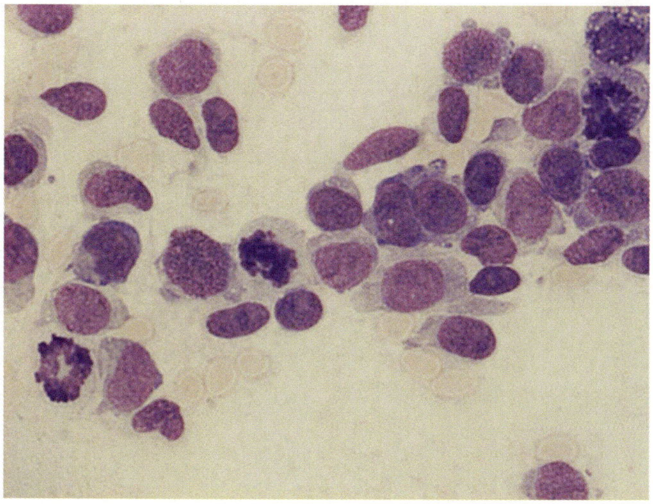
77g

Fig. 76. Extraskeletal myxoid chondrosarcoma. **a** In this case the smear is dominated by branching strands of loosely cohesive tumour cells. HE. Low magnification. **b** The myxoid matrix is best visualized in MGG. Small groups of rounded tumour cells are embedded in the matrix. MGG. Medium magnification. **c** Balls of tightly packed cells may be a typical feature and may resemble acinar structures in a mucinous carcinoma metastasis. MGG. Medium magnification. **d** The tumour cell population may focally consist of spindle cells. HE. Medium magnification.

Fig. 77. Synovial sarcoma. **a** The typical pattern under low power is a combination of dispersed cells and highly cellular branching tumour tissue fragments. HE. Low magnification. **b** Tumour cell nuclei in many cases of synovial sarcoma are relatively small, uniform, ovoid or rounded with bland chromatin and inconspicuous nucleoli. HE, oil. **c** Biphasic synovial sarcoma exhibiting an acinus-like structure. MGG. High magnification. **d** The tumour cells may be spindle-shaped and in these cases the differential diagnosis versus MPNST is difficult. HE. Medium magnification. **e** Cytokeratin-positive cells in a cell block preparation. **f** EMA is considered as a reliable marker for the epithelial differentiation in synovial sarcoma. Cell block preparation. **g** Poorly differentiated synovial sarcoma. Cellular and nuclear pleomorphism is marked. MGG. High magnification.

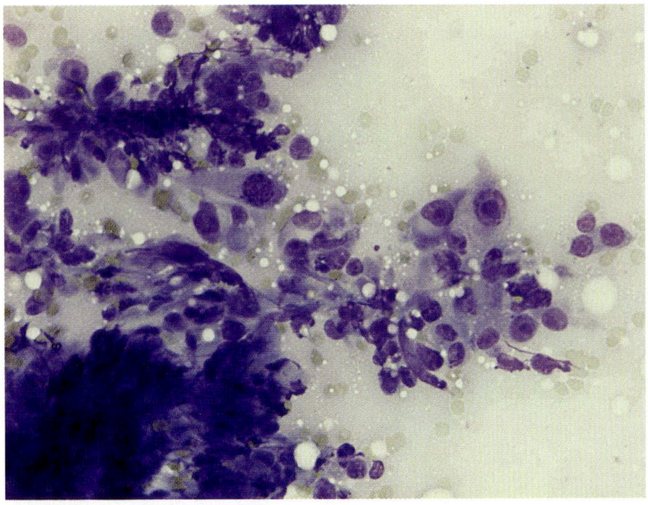

a

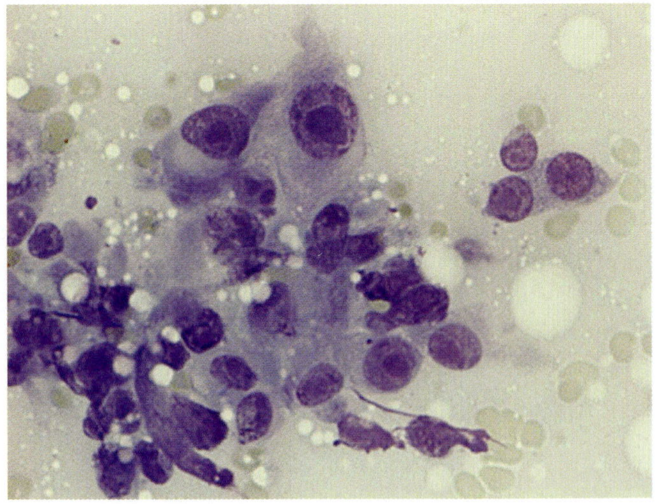

b

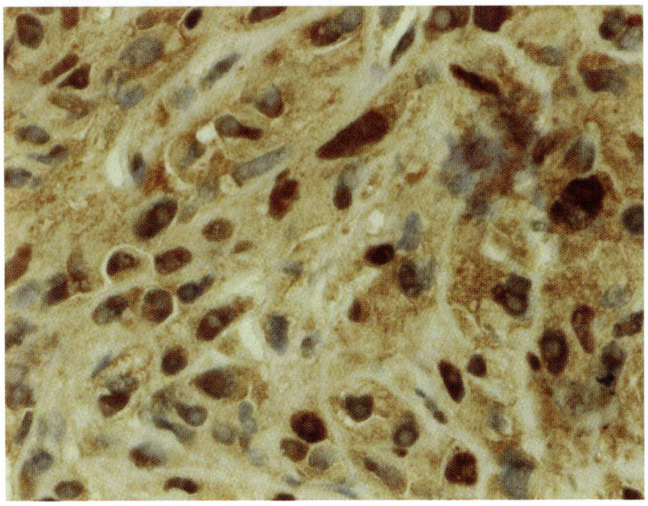

c

Fig. 78. Clear cell sarcoma. **a** A loosely cohesive cluster of tumour cells depicting a variable shape, rounded, elongated and polygonal. MGG. Medium magnification. **b** Prominent large nucleoli in many of the tumour cells. MGG. High magnification. **c** S-100 protein-positive tumour cells. Immunostaining, cell block preparation.

Cytological features of clear cell sarcoma (fig. 78a–c)

Mainly dispersed cells, but clusters of loosely cohesive cells may be present
Tumour cells are rounded, polygonal or spindly
Moderately abundant cytoplasm
Rounded or ovoid nuclei with large nucleoli
Moderate cellular pleomorphism
Occasionally scattered multinucleated tumour cells
Rarely pigmented tumour cells

Differential diagnosis

Melanoma (especially desmoplastic melanoma and metastatic melanoma)
MPNST
Carcinoma

Comment

As clear cell sarcoma is a deep-seated tumour, the distinction from primary melanoma is based on the tumour site. Clear cell sarcoma infiltrating the subcutis/cutis may be difficult to distinguish from desmoplastic melanoma, and soft tissue metastasis of melanoma is another pitfall. HMB45 and Melan A positivity is not seen in MPNST.

Chapter 6

Cytological Classification of Soft Tissue Tumours Based on the Principal Pattern

The majority of soft tissue tumours can be classified into one of the following five groups.

Pleomorphic Pattern

The typical features are a marked variation in cellular and nuclear size and shape and in case of sarcoma marked nuclear pleomorphism including atypical multinucleated tumour cells and prominent nucleoli.

Benign soft tissue tumours in this category are nodular fasciitis and pleomorphic lipoma.

Typical examples of sarcomas are pleomorphic sarcoma of the MFH type, pleomorphic leiomyosarcoma, pleomorphic liposarcoma and the less common pleomorphic MPNST and pleomorphic rhabdomyosarcoma.

Diagnostic pitfalls in this group are the pleomorphic malignant melanoma, anaplastic large cell carcinoma and ALCL (table 7).

Spindle Cell Pattern

The spindle cell pattern is characterized by a predominance of more or less atypical spindle cells with fusiform or ovoid nuclei and elongated uni- or bipolar cytoplasm. The cells are mostly arranged in sheets or fascicles, but dissociated cells are often present. A small population of larger rounded, polygonal or triangular cells with relatively abundant cytoplasm and nuclei of variable size and shape may be present in some sarcomas. Common examples of benign tumours are neurilemoma and desmoid fibromatosis, rare examples are deep-seated leiomyoma, spindle cell lipoma with a predominance of spindle cells and solitary fibrous tumour. Typical spindle cell sarcomas include the leiomyosarcoma, a subset of monophasic synovial sarcoma, MPNST and dermatofibrosarcoma protuberans and infrequently spindle cell GIST and fibrosarcoma (infantile and adult) (table 7).

Myxoid Pattern

The myxoid character is often noted already when the sample is smeared on the glass slides: a thick and viscous, more or less haemorrhagic fluid. Aspirates of myxoid tumours often look like droplets of glue. Under low power magnification there is an evident myxoid background matrix, blue or blue-violet, more or less fibrillary in MGG and faintly pink in HE and faintly green in Pap. The cellular pattern is variable: pleomorphic, spindly or round cells.

A myxoid pattern is common to several soft tissue tumours. Examples of benign tumours are intramuscular myxoma, many cases of nodular fasciitis, and the rare entities of OFMT, perineurioma, parachordoma and mixed tumour of soft tissue. The most common sarcomas are myxofibrosarcoma and myxoid liposarcoma, less common are low-grade fibromyxoid sarcoma and extraskeletal myxoid chondrosarcoma (table 8).

Small Round/Ovoid Cell Pattern

Smears are typically cellular and composed of small to medium-sized cells with rounded or ovoid nuclei and a variable amount of cytoplasm. The shape of the cells is variable: rounded, ovoid, fusiform or triangular. Nuclei are often bland and nucleoli small.

This pattern is shown mainly by sarcomas: extraskeletal ES/PNET, rhabdomyosarcoma (especially alveolar),

Table 7. Cytological evaluation of soft tissue tumours based on pleomorphic and spindle cell pattern

Tumour	Diagnostically important features	Ancillary tests	Notes
Pleomorphic pattern			
Nodular fasciitis	Marked pleomorphism in proliferating fibroblasts/myofibroblasts; ganglion cell-like cells; uniform chromatin structure	DNA ploidy analysis	Painful, tender, rapidly growing; most often spontaneous regression
MFH-type sarcoma	Marked pleomorphism, multinucleated (bizarre) tumour giant cells; mitoses (atypical); necrosis		
Pleomorphic leiomyosarcoma	Atypical cells with blunted/segmented nuclei; nuclei in tandem position	IC: desmin, SMA, caldesmon	
Pleomorphic MPNST	Atypical spindle cells with wavy, thin nuclei with pointed ends, coma-like nuclei	IC: S-100	
Pleomorphic rhabdomyosarcoma	Atypical rhabdomyoblast-like cells, triangular, rounded with eccentric nuclei and eosinophilic cytoplasm	IC: desmin, MyoD1, myoglobin	
Pitfalls			
Anaplastic carcinoma	Moulded clusters; 'owl's eye'	IC: cytokeratin	
Sarcomatous melanoma	Macronucleoli	IC: S-100, HMB45, Melan A	
Sarcomatous anaplastic large cell lymphoma	Reed-Sternberg-like cells; deep blue cytoplasm (MGG); presence of plasma cells, lymphocytes and histiocytes	IC: CD30, EMA, Alk1 Cytogenetic analysis	
Spindle cell pattern			
Neurilemoma	Predominantly tumour tissue fragments; indistinct cytoplasmic borders; fibrillary background; thin, wavy (comma-shaped) tapered nuclei; few dispersed cells	IC: S-100	Often sharp, radiating pain at needling; neurilemomas in extremities often fusiform at palpation and movable laterally but not craniocaudal
Desmoid	Runs, sheets or small groups of fibroblasts and fragments of cell-poor collagenous matrix; moderate pleomorphism in fibroblasts; occasionally muscle giant cells		Desmoid with prominent collagenous stroma firm to the needle and difficult to aspirate
Solitary fibrous tumour	Cell-tight irregular, three-dimensional tissue fragments mixed with dispersed cells; bland spindle cells	IC: CD34, CD99	
Deep leiomyoma	Tumour cells with cigar-shaped/blunted nuclei; segmented nuclei; moderate anisokaryosis; no mitoses	IC: desmin, SMA	
Leiomyosarcoma	Fascicles of more or less atypical spindle cells; cigar-shaped/blunted nuclei; segmented nuclei; nuclei in tandem position; scattered large atypical cells (stripped nuclei outside fascicles)	IC: desmin, SMA, caldesmon EM	

Table 7 (continued)

Tumour	Diagnostically important features	Ancillary tests	Notes
MPNST	Fascicles of atypical spindle cells with elongated, wavy nuclei with pointed ends; fibrillary background; comma-shaped nuclei; variable amount of dispersed cells	IC: S-100	
Monophasic synovial sarcoma	Mixture of cell-tight irregular, three-dimensional tissue fragment and dispersed cells with many stripped nuclei; often vascular network in fragments; bland nuclei but mitoses in fragments; mast cells	IC: EMA, cytokeratin, CD99 EM Cytogenetic analysis	Calcifications may be observed at radiographic investigation
Dermatofibrosarcoma protuberans	Mixture of cell-tight tissue, three-dimensional fragments and dispersed cells; moderate nuclear atypia; Touton-type giant cells and foam cells not present	IC: CD34	Cutaneous-subcutaneous tumour; often multinodular
Spindle cell GIST	No specific features; may mimick smooth muscle cells	IC: CD117, CD34	Abdominal tumour
Adult fibrosarcoma	Sheets, fascicles of atypical spindle cells		Diagnosis of exclusion
Pitfalls			
Squamous cell carcinoma, spindle cell type		IC: cytokeratins	
Spindle cell malignant melanoma		IC: HMB45, Melan A	

Table 8. Cytological evaluation of soft tissue tumours based on pattern: myxoid pattern

Tumour	Diagnostically important features	Ancillary tests	Notes
Intramuscular myxoma	Poor cellularity; small cell clusters and dispersed cells; cells with long thin bipolar cytoplasmic processes and ovoid or elongated bland nuclei; occasionally individual vessel fragments and 'muscle giant cells'		
OFMT	Mixture of dissociated cells and cell clusters; occasionally acinar-like structures; rounded nuclei in cytoplasm-rich cells	IC: S-100, SMA	Subcutaneous tumour Thick fibrous capsula often with bone trabeculae
Perineurioma	Elongated cells with thin cytoplasmic processes; rounded, ovoid or fusiform nuclei; moderate anisokaryosis; stripped nuclei	IC: EMA	Extremely rare
Parachordoma	Variable cellular morphology: rounded, elongated, polygonal cells; rounded or ovoid nuclei; cytoplasmic vacuolation; moderate anisokaryosis (chordoma-like cytology)	IC: S-100, cytokeratin	Extremely rare
Mixed tumour of soft tissue	Salivary pleomorphic adenoma-like cytology	IC: cytokeratin, S-100, SMA, GFAP	Site important for diagnosis; subcutaneous tumours difficult to distinguish from chondroid syringoma

Table 8 (continued)

Tumour	Diagnostically important features	Ancillary tests	Notes
Myxofibrosarcoma	Curved vessel fragments in myxoid background; low-grade tumours predominantly spindly with moderate atypia; high grade tumours pleomorphic		
Low-grade fibromyxoid sarcoma	Slight to moderate atypia in constitutional spindle cells; occasional vessel fragments in myxoid background		Difficult to distinguish from low-grade myxofibrosarcoma
EMC	Variable arrangement of cells: cell balls, branching strands, clusters; chondroblastoma-like nuclei (coffee bean nuclei); almost never cartilage-like fragments	IC: S-100 Cytogenetic analysis	
Pitfalls			
Myxoid malignant melanoma		IC: HMB45, Melan A	

Table 9. Cytological evaluation of soft tissue tumours based on pattern: small round ovoid cell pattern

Tumour	Diagnostically important features	Ancillary tests	Notes
Glomus tumour	Presence of myxoid background matrix; lesional cells with rounded, ovoid, bland nuclei; presence of spindle cells	IC: SMA	Intensive pain at needling
Neuroblastoma	Dispersed cells and clusters; stripped nuclei; neuropil background; small moulded clusters, occasional rosettes; in preserved cells long thin cytoplasmic processes connecting cells; dark irregular nuclei	IC: NSE, chromogranin, synaptophysin EM	
ES/PNET family; classic ES	Double cell population large light and small dark cells; large cells with abundant cytoplasm with vacuoles and clear spaces; bland nuclear morphology, inconspicuous nucleoli	IC: CD99 EM Cytogenetic analysis	
ES/PNET family; PNET	Occasional rosettes; small unipolar cytoplasmic processes; moderate pleomorphism	IC: CD99, NSE, chromogranin EM Cytogenetic analysis	
Alveolar rhabdomyosarcoma	Rounded, pear-shaped or triangular myoblast-like cells; eosinophilic cytoplasm; occasionally multinucleated giant cells with numerous small nuclei	IC: desmin, MyoD1 EM Cytogenetic analysis	
Desmoplastic small round cell tumour	Dispersed cells and loosely cohesive clusters; scant cytoplasm; inconspicuous nucleoli; occasionally stromal fibroblasts	IC: cytokeratin, desmin, NSE Cytogenetic analysis	Predominantly abdominal tumour
Poorly differentiated areas in synovial sarcoma	Mixture of cell-tight irregular, three-dimensional tissue fragments and dispersed cells with stripped nuclei; vessel network in fragments; preserved cells small with rounded ES-like nuclei	IC: EMA, cytokeratin, CD99 EM Cytogenetic analysis	
Pitfalls			
Small cell carcinoma		IC: cytokeratin	
Lymphoblastic lymphoma		IC: CD3, CD79a; CD10, Tdt	
Small cell melanoma		IC: S-100, HMB45, Melan A	

Table 10. Cytological evaluation of soft tissue tumours based on pattern: epithelioid cell pattern

Tumour	Diagnostically important features	Ancillary tests	Notes
Granular cell tumour	Stripped nuclei and granular background; abundant cytoplasm, indistinct cytoplasmic borders; granulated cytoplasm; predominantly small nuclei	IC: S-100, NSE EM	
Adult rhabdomyoma	Abundant eosinophilic, granulated cytoplasm; cytoplasmic vacuolation; small nuclei with prominent nucleoli	IC: desmin, myoglobin	
Paraganglioma	Acinar/follicle-like structures; moderate pleomorphism; red-granulated cytoplasm	IC: NSE, chromogranin EM	
Epithelioid sarcoma	Rounded, polygonal, spindly tumour cells; large nucleoli; admixture of lymphocytes, plasma cells, histiocytes, granuloma-like structures; necrosis	IC: cytokeratin, EMA, CD34	Ulceration may be seen in subcutaneous tumours; inflammatory cells may predominate
Clear cell sarcoma	Predominantly dispersed cells; round, polygonal tumour cells; rounded nuclei with prominent nucleoli	IC: S-100, HMB45, Melan A	
Alveolar soft part sarcoma	Moderately abundant granular cytoplasm; binucleated, multinucleated cells; rounded nuclei with prominent nucleoli; stripped nuclei	IC: muscle specific actin, SMA, desmin EM	
Malignant extrarenal rhabdoid tumour	Variable cellular shape; eccentric nuclei; prominent nucleoli; cytoplasmic paranuclear inclusions	IC: cytokeratin, NSE	
Pitfalls			
Malignant melanoma		IC: HMB45, Melan A	Site of tumour important versus clear cell sarcoma
Carcinoma		IC: cytokeratins EM	

neuroblastoma, pure round cell liposarcoma, most monophasic synovial sarcoma and desmoplastic small round cell malignant tumour. The main diagnostic pitfalls are small cell carcinoma, non-Hodgkin's lymphoma and small cell malignant melanoma (table 9).

Epithelioid Cell Pattern

The epithelioid cell pattern is created by cells with epithelioid features: rounded or polygonal cells with distinct cytoplasmic borders, rather abundant cytoplasm, and rounded, ovoid or irregular nuclei. Nucleoli are often prominent. The tumour cells are arranged in groups, tight clusters or are dissociated. Stripped nuclei are a common finding. Most tumours in this group are rare and infrequent targets for needling. Typical examples of benign tumours are granular cell tumour, adult rhabdomyoma and paraganglioma and among the sarcomas epithelioid sarcoma, clear cell sarcoma, alveolar soft part sarcoma, malignant rhabdoid tumour and epithelioid cell GIST. Diagnostic pitfalls include carcinoma and malignant melanoma (table 10).

It is not possible to classify all soft tissue tumours into these five groups. In most benign adipose tumours large fat cells predominate and vascular tumours may appear as examples of either the pleomorphic pattern, the spindle cell pattern or the epithelioid cell pattern.

Summary and Conclusions

FNA used in the primary diagnostic workup of soft tissue tumours has a number of advantages over open biopsy and core needle biopsy. In most sarcomas where primary surgery is the treatment, FNA diagnosis is accurate enough for the planning of the surgical intervention. In those sarcomas where neoadjuvant therapy followed by surgery is the treatment of choice, the FNA diagnosis must be equivalent to histology with regard to histotype and malignancy grading. In these cases routine cytological examination often has to be supplemented with ancillary diagnostics.

The optimal use of FNA as a pretreatment diagnostic tool requires the referral of patients to multidisciplinary centres where the cytopathologist is a member of the team and a close cooperation between the cytopathologist and surgeon [3].

References

1 Kempson RL, Fletcher CDM, Evans HL, Hendrickson MR, Sibley RK: Atlas of Tumor Pathology. Tumors of the Soft Tissues. Washington, Armed Forces Institute of Pathology, 2001.
2 Weiss SW, Goldblum JR: Soft Tissue Tumors, ed 4. St Louis, Mosby, 2001.
3 Rydholm A: Centralisation of soft tissue sarcoma: The Southern Sweden Experience. Acta Orthop Scand 1997;68(suppl 273):4–8.
4 Domanski HA, Carlén B, Gustafson P, Rydholm A, Åkerman M: Needle core biopsy performed by the cytopathologist: A technique to complement fine needle aspiration of musculoskeletal tumors. 28th European Congress of Cytology, Antwerp, 2002.
5 Miralles T, Gosalbez F, Menendez P, Astudillo A, Torre C, Buesa J: Fine needle aspiration cytology of soft-tissue lesions. Acta Cytol 1986; 30:671–677.
6 Maitra A, Ashfaq R, Saboorian MH, Lindberg G, Gokaslan S: The role of fine-needle aspiration biopsy in the primary diagnosis of mesenchymal lesions: A community hospital-based experience. Cancer 2000; 90/3:178–185.
7 Wakely P, Kneisl J: Soft tissue aspiration cytopathology. Diagnostic accuracy and limitations. Cancer 2000;5:292–298.
8 Kilpatrick SE, Capellari JO, Bos GD, Gold SH, Ward WG: Is fine-needle aspiration biopsy a practical alternative to open biopsy for the primary diagnosis of sarcoma? Am J Clin Pathol 2001;115:59–68.
9 Åkerman M: The cytology of soft tissue tumours. Acta Orthop Scand 1997;65(suppl 273):54–59.
10 Brosjö O, Bauer HCP, Kriecbergs A: Fine needle aspiration biopsy of soft tissue tumours. Acta Orthop Scand 1994;65 (suppl 256):108–109.
11 Åkerman M: Fine-needle aspiration cytology of soft tissue sarcoma: Benefits and limitations. Sarcoma 1998;2:155–161.
12 Liu K, Layfield L, Coogan A, Ballo M, Bentz J, Dodge R: Diagnostic accuracy in fine-needle aspiration of soft tissue and bone lesions. Influence of clinical history and experience. Am J Clin Pathol 1999;111: 632–640.
13 Dahl I, Åkerman M: Nodular fasciitis. A correlative cytologic and histologic study of 13 cases. Acta Cytol 1981;25:91–101.
14 Lundgren L, Kindblom L-G, Willems J, Falkmer U, Angervall L: Proliferative myositis and fasciitis. A light and electron microscopic, cytologic, DNA-cytometric and immunohistochemical study. APMIS 1992; 100:437–448.
15 Rööser B, Herrlin K, Rydholm A, Åkerman M: Pseudomalignant myositis ossificans. Clinical, radiologic and cytologic diagnosis in 5 cases. Acta Orthop Scand 1989;60:457–460.
16 Walaas L, Kindblom L-G: Lipomatous tumors. A correlative cytologic and histologic study of 27 tumors examined by fine needle aspiration cytology. Hum Pathol 1985;16:6–18
17 Åkerman M, Rydholm A: Aspiration cytology of lipomatous tumors. A 10 year experience at an Orthopedic Oncology Center. Diagn Cytopathol 1987;3:295–302.
18 Lemos MM, Kindblom L-G, Meiss-Kindblom JM, Remotti F, Ryd W, Gunterberg B, Willén H: Fine-needle aspiration characteristics of hibernoma. Cancer 2001;93:206–210.
19 Domanski HA, Carlén B, Jonsson K, Mertens F, Åkerman M: Distinct cytologic features of spindle cell lipoma. A cytologic-histologic study with clinical, radiologic, electron microscopic, and cytogenetic correlations. Cancer 2001;93:381–389.
20 Dahl I, Hagmar B, Idvall I: Benign solitary neurilemoma. A correlative cytological and histological study of 28 cases. Acta Pathol Microbiol Immunol Scand 1984;92:91–101.
21 Resnick JM, Fanning CV, Caraway NP, Varma DGK, Johnson M: Percutaneous needle biopsy diagnosis of benign neurogenic neoplasms. Diagn Cytopathol 1997;16: 17–25.
22 Mooney EE, Layfield LL, Dodd LG: Fine-needle aspiration of neural lesions. Diagn Cytopathol 1999;20:1–5.
23 Wieczorek TJ, Krane JF, Domanski HA, Åkerman M, Carlén B, Misdraji J, Granter SR: Cytologic findings in granular cell tumors with emphasis on the diagnosis of malignant granular cell tumor by fine-needle aspiration biopsy. Cancer 2001;93:398–408.
24 Åkerman M, Rydholm A: Aspiration cytology of intramuscular myxoma. A comparative clinical, cytologic and histologic study of ten cases. Acta Cytol 1983;27:505–510.
25 Domanski HA: Cytologic features of angioleiomyoma. Cytologic-histologic study of 10 cases. Diagn Cytopathol 2002;27:161–166.
26 Walaas L, Angervall L, Hagmar B, Säve-Söderberg J: Correlative cytologic and histologic study of malignant fibrous histiocytoma: An analysis of 40 cases examined by fine-needle aspiration cytology. Diagn Cytopathol 1986;2:46–54.
27 Berardo M, Powers C, Wakely P, Almeida MO, Frable W: Fine needle aspiration cytopathology of MFH. Cancer 1997;81:228–237.
28 Merck C, Hagmar B: Myxofibrosarcoma. A correlative cytologic and histologic study of 13 cases examined by fine needle aspiration. Acta Cytol 1980;24:137–144.
29 Kilpatrick SE, Ward WG: Myxofibrosarcoma of soft tissues: Cytomorphologic analysis of a series. Diagn Cytopathol 1999;20:6–9.
30 Dahl I, Hagmar B, Angervall L: Leiomyosarcoma of the soft tissue. A correlative cytological and histological study of 11 cases. Acta Pathol Microbiol Immunol Scand 1981;89:285–291.
31 Nemanqani D, Mourad WA: Cytomorphologic features of fine-needle aspiration of liposarcoma. Diagn Cytopathol 1999;20:67–69.
32 Szadowska A, Lasota J: Fine needle aspiration cytology of myxoid liposarcoma: A study of 18 tumors. Cytopathology 1993;4:99–106.
33 McGee RS Jr, Ward WG, Kilpatrick SE: Malignant peripheral nerve sheath tumor: A fine-needle aspiration biopsy study. Diagn Cytopathol 1997;17:298–305.
34 Klijanienko J, Caillaud J-M, Lagacé R, Viehl P: Cytohistologic correlations of 24 malignant peripheral nerve sheath tumor (MPNST) in 17 patients: The Institut Curie Experience. Diagn Cytopathol 2002;27:103–108.
35 Kilpatrick SE, Teot LA, Stanley MW, Ward WG, Savage PD, Geisinger KR: Fine-needle aspiration biopsy of synovial sarcoma. A cytomorphologic analysis of primary, recurrent, and metastatic tumors. Am J Clin Pathol 1996; 106:769–775.
36 Åkerman M, Willén H, Carlén B: Fine needle aspiration (FNA) of synovial sarcoma – A comparative histological-cytological study of 15 cases, including immunohistochemical, electron microscopic and cytogenetic examination and DNA-ploidy analysis. Cytopathology 1996;7:187–200.
37 Ryan MR, Stastny JF, Wakely PE: The cytopathology of synovial sarcoma: A study of six cases, with emphasis on architecture and histopathologic correlation. Cancer 1998;84: 42–49.

38 Klijanienko J, Caillaud J-M, Lagacé R, Viehl P: Cytohistologic correlations in 56 synovial sarcomas in 36 patients: The Institut Curie experience. Diagn Cytopathol 2002;27: 96–102.
39 Akhtar M, Ali M, Bakry M, Hug M, Sackey K: Fine-needle aspiration biopsy diagnosis of rhabdomyosarcoma. Cytologic, histologic and ultrastructural correlations. Diagn Cytopathol 1992;8:465–474.
40 Atahan S, Aksu Ö, Ekinci C: Cytologic diagnosis and subtyping of rhabdomyosarcoma. Cytopathology 1998;9:389–397.
41 de Almeida M, Statsny JF, Wakely PE, Frable WJ: Fine needle aspiration biopsy of childhood rhabdomyosarcoma: Re-evaluation of the cytologic criteria for diagnosis. Diagn Cytopathol 1994;11:231–236.
42 Seidal T, Mark K, Hagmar B, Angervall L: Alveolar rhabdomyosarcoma: A cytogenetic and correlated cytological and histological study. Acta Pathol Microbiol Immunol Scand 1982;90:345–354.
43 de Jong ASH, van Kessel-van Vark M, van Heerde P: Fine-needle aspiration biopsy diagnosis of rhabdomyosarcoma: An immunocytochemical study. Acta Cytol 1987;31:573–577.
44 Seidal T, Walaas L, Kindblom L-G, Angervall L: Cytology of embryonal rhabdomyosarcoma: Cytologic, light microscopic, electron microscopic and immunohistochemical study of six cases. Diagn Cytopathol 1988;4:242–299.
45 Akhtar M, Ali M, Sackey K, Sabbah R, Bakry M: Aspiration cytology of neuroblastoma: Light microscopy with transmission and scanning electron microscopic correlations. Diagn Cytopathol 1988;4:323–327.
46 Åkerman M, Carlén B: Diagnosis of neuroblastoma in fine needle aspirates. Acta Orthop Scand 1997;68(suppl 274):72.
47 Liu K, Layfield LJ: Cytomorphologic features of angiosarcoma on fine needle aspiration biopsy. Acta Cytol 1999;43:407–415.
48 Boucher LD, Swanson PE, Stanley MW, Silverman JF, Raab SS, Geisinger KR: Cytology of angiosarcoma. Findings in fourteen fine-needle aspiration biopsy specimens and one pleural fluid specimen. Am J Clin Pathol 2000; 114:210–219.
49 Minimo C, Zakowski M, Lin O: Cytologic findings of malignant vascular neoplasms: A study of twenty-four cases. Diagn Cytopathol 2002; 26:349–355.
50 Shabb N, Fanning C, Dekmezian R: Fine needle aspiration cytology of alveolar soft part sarcoma. Diagn Cytopathol 1991;7:293–298.
51 Persson S, Willems JS, Kindblom L-G, Angervall L: Alveolar soft part sarcoma. An immunohistochemical, cytologic and electron microscopic study and quantitative DNA analysis. Virchows Arch A Pathol Anat Histopathol 1988;412:499–513.
52 Caraway NP, Fanning C, Wojcik EM, Staerkel GA, Benjamin RS, Ordonez NG: Cytology of malignant melanoma of soft parts: Fine-needle aspirates and exfoliative specimens. Diagn Cytopathol 1993;9:632–638.
53 Powers CN, Hurt MA, Frable W: Fine-needle aspiration biopsy: Dermatofibrosarcoma protuberans. Diagn Cytopathol 1993;9:145–150.
54 Domanski HA, Gustafson P: Cytologic features of primary, recurrent and metastatic dermatofibrosarcoma protuberans. Cancer 2002;96: 351–361.
55 Cardillo M, Zakowski MF, Lin O: Fine-needle aspiration of epithelioid sarcoma: Cytology findings in nine cases. Cancer 2001;93: 246–251.
56 Zeppa P, Errico ME, Palombini L: Epithelioid sarcoma: Report of two cases diagnosed by fine-needle aspiration biopsy with immunohistochemical correlation. Diagn Cytopathol 1999; 21:405–408.
57 Åkerman M, Willén H: Critical review on the role of fine needle aspiration in soft tissue tumors. Pathol Case Rev 1998;3:111–117.
58 Ward W, Savage P, Boles C, Kilpatrick S: Fine needle aspiration biopsy of sarcomas and related tumors. Cancer Control 2001;8: 232–238.
59 Domanski HA, Gustafson P, Åkerman M: Fine needle aspiration of musculoskeletal tumors: The experience from an orthopedic tumor center showing diagnostic value of cell block preparation. Acta Cytol 2002; 1(suppl):115.
60 Nordgren H, Åkerman M: Electron microscopy of fine needle aspiration biopsy from soft tissue tumors. Acta Cytol 1982;26: 179–188.
61 Kindblom L-G, Walaas L, Widehn S: Ultrastructural studies in the preoperative cytologic diagnosis of soft-tissue tumors. Semin Diagn Pathol 1986;3:317–344.
62 Åkerman M, Killander D, Rydholm A: Aspiration of musculoskeletal tumors for cytodiagnosis and DNA analysis. Acta Orthop Scand 1987;58:523–528.
63 Fernö M, Baldetorp B, Åkerman M: Flow cytometric DNA ploidy analysis of soft tissue sarcoma. A comparative study of preoperative fine needle aspirate and postoperative fresh tissue and archival material. Anal Quant Cytol Histol 1990;12:251–258.
64 Åkerman M, Dreinhöfer K, Rydholm A, Willén H, Mertens F, Mitelman F, Mandahl N: Cytogenetic studies on fine-needle aspiration samples from osteosarcoma and Ewing's sarcoma. Diagn Cytopathol 1995;15:17–22.
65 Nilsson G, Ming MD, Wejde J, Kanter L, Karlén J, Tani E, Kreicbergs A, Larsson O: Reverse transcriptase polymerase chain reaction on fine needle aspirates for rapid detection of translocations in synovial sarcoma. Acta Cytol 1998;42:1317–1324.
66 Fröstad B: Fine needle aspiration cytology in diagnosis and management of childhood small round cell tumours. Thesis, Stockholm, 2000.
67 Udaykumar AM, Sundareshan TS, Appaji L, Biswas S, Mukherje G: Rhabdomyosarcoma: Cytogenetics of five cases using fine-needle aspiration samples and review of the literature. Ann Genet 2002;45:33–37.
68 Bjerkehagen B, Dietrich C, Reed W, Micci F, Saeter G, Berner A, Nesland JM, Heim S: Extraskeletal myxoid chondrosarcoma: Multimodal diagnosis and identification of a new cytogenetic subgroup characterized by t(9;17). Virchows Arch 1999;435:524–530.
69 Talwar MB, Misra K, Marya SHS, Dev G: Fine-needle aspiration cytology of lipoblastoma. Acta Cytol 1993;37:563–565.
70 Gisselsson D, Domanski HA, Höglund M, Carlén B, Mertens F, Willén H: Unique cytologic features and chromosome aberrations in chondroid lipoma: A case report based on fine-needle aspiration cytology, histopathology, electron microscopy, chromosome banding, and molecular cytogenetics. Am J Surg Pathol 1999;23:1300–1304.
71 Thomson TA, Horsman D, Bainbridge TC: Cytogenetic and cytologic features of chondroid lipoma of soft tissue. Mod Pathol 1999; 12:88–91.
72 Prahlow JA, Loggie BV, Capellari JO, Scharling ES, Teot LA, Iskander SS: Extra-adrenal myelolipoma: Report of two cases. South Med J 1995;88:639–643.
73 Weiss SW: Histological Typing of Soft Tissue Tumours. World Health Organisation International Histological Classification of Tumours. New York, Springer, 1994.
74 Stanley M, Skoog L, Tani E, Horwitz C: Spontaneous resolution of nodular fasciitis following diagnosis by fine needle aspiration. Acta Cytol 1991;35:616–617.
75 Willén H, Åkerman M: Fine needle aspiration of nodular fasciitis – No need for surgery. Acta Orthop Scand 1995;66 (suppl 265):54–55.
76 Willén H, Carlén B, Rydholm A, Gustafson P: Solitary fibrous tumor of the soft tissue. Acta Orthop Scand 1999;70(suppl 289):31–32.
77 Pisharodi LR, Cary D, Bernacki EG Jr: Elastofibroma dorsi: Diagnostic problems and pitfalls. Diagn Cytopathol 1994;10: 242–244.
78 Mojica WD, Kuntzman T: Elastofibroma dorsi: Elaboration of cytologic features and review of its pathogenesis. Diagn Cytopathol 2000;23: 393–396.
79 Evans HL: Low grade fibromyxoid sarcoma. A report of 12 cases. Am J Surg Pathol 1993; 17:595–600.
80 Goodlad JR, Mentzel T, Fletcher CD: Low grade fibromyxoid sarcoma: Clinicopathological analysis of eleven new cases in support of a distinct entity. Histopathology 1995;26: 229–237.
81 Lindberg GM, Maitra A, Gokasian ST, Saboorian MH, Albores-Saavedra JA: Low grade fibromyxoid sarcoma. Fine-needle aspiration cytology with histologic, cytogenetic, immunohistochemical and ultrastructural correlation. Cancer 1999;87:75–82.
82 Pereira S, Tani E, Skoog L: Diagnosis of fibromatosis colli by fine needle aspiration. Cytopathology 1999;1:25–29.
83 Jadushing IH: Fine needle aspiration cytology of fibrous hamartoma of infancy. Acta Cytol 1997;41(suppl 4):1391–1393.
84 Meis-Kindblom J, Bjerkehagen B, Böhling T, Domanski H, Halvorsen TB, Larsson O, Lilleng P, Myhre-Jensen O, Stenwig E, Virolainen M, Willén H, Åkerman M, Kindblom L-G: Morphologic review of 1000 soft tissue sarcomas from the Scandinavian Sarcoma Group (SSG) Register. The peer-review committee experience. Acta Orthop Scand 1999;70(suppl 285):18–26.

85 Fletcher CDM, Gustafson P, Rydholm A, Willén H, Åkerman M: Clinicopathologic re-evaluation of 100 malignant fibrous histiocytomas: Prognostic relevance of subclassification. J Clin Oncol 2001;19:3045–3050.
86 Hollowood K, Fletcher CDM: Malignant fibrous histiocytoma. Morphologic pattern or pathologic entity? Semin Diagn Pathol 1995; 12:210–220.
87 Fletcher CD, Kilpatrick SE, Mentzel T: The difficulty in predicting behaviour of smooth-muscle tumors in deep soft tissue. Am J Surg Pathol 1995;19:116–117.
88 Bondesson L, Andreasson L: Aspiration cytology of adult rhabdomyoma. Acta Cytol 1986;30:679–682.
89 Domanski HA, Dawiskiba S: Adult rhabdomyoma in fine needle aspiration. A report of two cases. Acta Cytol 2000;44:223–226.
90 Tsokos M, Webber BL, Parham DM: Rhabdomyosarcoma: A new classification scheme related to prognosis. Arch Pathol Lab Med 1992;116:847–856.
91 Coffin CM: The new international rhabdomyosarcoma classification, its progenitors, and considerations beyond morphology. Adv Anat Pathol 1997;4:1–16.
92 Åkerman M, Carlén B: Fine needle aspiration cytology of rhabdomyosarcoma. Is a reliable type diagnosis possible to render. A retrospective study of 23 cases. Acta Orthop Scand 1996;67(suppl 272):55.
93 Ryd W, Mugel S, Ayyash K: Ancient neurilemoma. A pitfall in the cytologic diagnosis of soft tissue tumors. Diagn Cytopathol 1988;2: 244–247.
94 Dodd L, Marom EM, Dash R, Matthews MR, McLendon RE: Fine needle aspiration of 'ancient schwannoma'. Diagn Cytopathol 1999;20:307–311.
95 Henke AC, Salomao DR, Hughes JH: Cellular schwannoma mimics a sarcoma: An example of a potential pitfall in aspiration cytodiagnosis. Diagn Cytopathol 1999;20: 312–316.
96 Housini I, Dabbs DJ: Fine needle aspiration cytology of perineurioma. Report of a case with histologic, immunohistochemical and ultrastructural studies. Acta Cytol 1990;34: 420–424.
97 Layfield LJ, Mooney EE, Dodd LG: Not by blood alone: Diagnosis of hemangioma by fine needle aspiration. Diagn Cytopathol 1998;19:250–254.
98 Fletcher CD: Hemangiopericytoma – A dying breed? Reappraisal of an 'entity' and its variants: A hypothesis. Curr Diagn Pathol 1994;1:19–25.
99 Nappi O, Ritter JH, Pettinato G, Wick MR: Hemangiopericytoma: Histologic pattern or clinicopathologic entity? Semin Diagn Pathol 1995;12:221–232.
100 Handa V, Palfa A, Mohan H, Punja RPS: Aspiration cytology of glomus tumor. A case report. Acta Cytol 2001;45:1073–1076.
101 Hood IC, Qizilbash AH, Young JE, Archibald SD: Fine needle aspiration biopsy cytology of paraganglioma. Cytologic, light microscopic and ultrastructural studies of three cases. Acta Cytol 1983;27:651–657.
102 Gonzales-Campora R, Otel-Salaverri C, Panea-Flores D, Lerma-Puertas E, Galera Davidsson H: Fine needle aspiration cytology of paraganglionic tumors. Acta Cytol 1988;32:386–390.
103 Das DK, Gupta AK, Chowdhury V, Satsangi DL, Tyagi S, Mohan JC, Khan VA, Malhotra V: Fine-needle aspiration diagnosis of carotid body tumor: Report of a case and review of experience with cytologic features in four cases. Diagn Cytopathol 1997;17: 143–147.
104 Dodd LG, Nelson RC, Mooney EE, Gottfried M: Fine-needle aspiration of gastrointestinal stromal tumors. Am J Clin Pathol 1998; 109:439–443.
105 Li SQ, O'Leary TJ, Buchner SB, Przygodzki RM, Sobin LH, Erozon YS, Rosenthal DL: Fine needle aspiration of gastrointestinal stromal tumors. Acta Cytol 2001;45:9–17.
106 Rader A, Avery A, Wait C, McGreevey L, Faigal D, Heinrich M: Fine-needle aspiration biopsy diagnosis of gastrointestinal stromal tumor using morphology, immunocytochemistry, and mutational analysis of c-kit. Cancer 2001;93:269–275.
107 Fröstad B, Tani E, Kogner P, Maeda S, Björck O, Skoog L: The clinical use of fine needle aspiration cytology for diagnosis and management of children with neuroblastic tumours. Eur J Cancer 1998;34: 529–536.
108 Akhtar M, Ali MA, Abbah R: Aspiration cytology of Ewing's sarcoma. Cancer 1985; 56:2051–2060.
109 Dahl I, Åkerman M: Ewing's sarcoma of bone. A cytological and histological study of 14 cases. Acta Pathol Microbiol Immunol Scand 1986;94:363–369.
110 Bakhos R, Andrey J, Bhoopalam N, Jensen J, Reyes C: Fine-needle aspiration cytology of extraskeletal Ewing's sarcoma. Diagn Cytopathol 1998;18:137–140.
111 Renshaw A, Perez-Atayde P, Fletcher J, Granter S: Cytology of typical and atypical Ewing's sarcoma/PNET. Am J Clin Pathol 1996;106:620–624.
112 Silverman JF, Berns L, Tate Holbrook C: Fine needle aspiration cytology of primitive neuroectodermal tumors. A report of three cases. Acta Cytol 1992;36:543–550.
113 González-Kámpora R, Otal-Salaverri C, Flores PP, Hevia-Vazques A, Pascual AG, Diez VSM: Fine needle aspiration of peripheral neuroepithelioma of soft tissues. Acta Cytol 1992;36:152–158.
114 Nicol K, Wars W, Savage PD, Kilpatrick S: Fine-needle aspiration biopsy of skeletal versus extraskeletal osteosarcoma. Cancer 1998;84:176–185.
115 Åkerman M, Domanski HA: Fine needle aspiration (FNA) of bone tumors with special emphasis on the definitive treatment of primary malignant bone tumors based on FNA. Curr Diagn Pathol 1998;5:82–92.
116 Nielsen GP, O'Conell JX, Rosenberg AE: Intramuscular myxoma: A clinicopathologic study of 51 cases with emphasis on hypercellular and hypervascular variants. Am J Surg Pathol 1998;22:1222–1227.
117 Catroppo J, Olesnicky L, Ringer P, Goldenkranz R, Casas V, Wright T: Intramuscular low-grade myxoid neoplasm with recurrent porential (cellular myxoma) of the lower extremity: Case report with cytohistologic correlation and review of the literature. Diagn Cytopathol 2002;26:301–305.
118 Enzinger FM, Weiss SW, Liang CY: Ossifying fibromyxoid tumor of soft parts. A clinicopathologic analysis of 59 cases. Am J Surg Pathol 1989;13:817–827.
119 Kilpatrick SE, Ward MG, Mozes M, Miettinen M, Fukanga F, Fletcher CD: Atypical and malignant variants of ossifying fibromyxoid tumor: Clinicopathologic analysis of six cases. Am J Surg Pathol 1995;19: 1039–1046.
120 Lax S, Langsteger W: Ossifying fibromyxoid tumor misdiagnosed as follicular neoplasia. A case report. Acta Cytol 1997;41:1261–1264.
121 Kilpatrick SE, Hitchcock MG, Kraus MD, Calonje E, Fletcher CD: Mixed tumor and myoepithelioma of soft tissue: A clinicopathologic study of 19 cases with a unifying concept. Am J Surg Pathol 1997;21:13–22.
122 Fisher C, Miettinen M: Parachordoma: A clinicopathologic and immunohistochemical study of four cases of an unusual soft tissue neoplasm. Ann Diagn Pathol 1997;1:3–10.
123 Folpe AL, Agoff SN, Willis J, Weiss SW: Parachordoma is immunohistochemically and cytogenetically distinct from axial chordoma and extraskeletal myxoid chondrosarcoma. Am J Surg Pathol 1999;23: 1059–1067.
124 Ordonez NG: Desmoplastic small round cell tumor. II. An ultrastructural and immunohistochemical study with emphasis on new immunohistochemical markers. Am J Surg Pathol 1998;22:1314–1327.
125 Caraway NP, Fanning CV, Amato RJ, Ordonez NG, Katz RL: Fine-needle aspiration of intra-abdominal desmoplastic small cell tumor. Diagn Cytopathol 1993;9: 465–470.
126 Ali SZ, Nicol TL, Port J, Ford G: Intraabdominal desmoplastic small round cell tumor: Cytopathologic finding in two cases. Diagn Cytopathol 1998;18:449–452.
127 Ferlicot C, Coue O, Gilbert E, Beuzeboc P, Servois V, Klijanienko J, Delattre O, Vielh P: Intraabdominal desmoplastic small round cell tumor: Report of a case with fine needle aspiration, cytologic diagnosis and molecular confirmation. Acta Cytol 2001;45:617–621.
128 Akhtar M, Kfoury H, Haider A, Sackey K, Ali MA: Fine-needle aspiration biopsy diagnosis of extrarenal malignant rhabdoid tumor. Diagn Cytopathol 1994;11:271–276.
129 Pogacnik A, Zidar N: Malignant rhabdoid tumor of the liver diagnosed by fine needle aspiration cytology. A case report. Acta Cytol 1997;41:539–543.
130 Guillou L, Wadden C, Coindre JM, Krausz T, Fletcher CD: 'Proximal-type' epithelioid sarcoma, a distinctive aggressive neoplasm showing rhabdoid features. Clinicopathologic, immunohistochemical, and ultrastructural study of a series. Am J Surg Pathol 1997;21: 130–146.

131 Goh Y-W, Spagnolo DV, Platten M, Caterina P, Fisher C, Oliveira AM, Nascimento AG: Extraskeletal myxoid chondrosarcoma: A light microscopic, immunohistochemical, ultrastructural and immuno-ultrastructural study indicating neuroendocrine differentiation. Histopathology 2001;39:514–524.

132 Willen H, Lemos M, Ryd W, Meis-Kindblom JM, Kindblom LG: Extraskeletal myxoid chondrosarcoma. A cytologic and histologic correlation. 1st Italian/Scandinavian Sarcoma Group Meeting-ISG/SSG. Acta Orthop Scand 2000;http://home.pi.se/actaorthopscand/pages/framabst.html.p33.

133 Örndal C, Carlén B, Åkerman M, Willén H, Mandahl N, Heim S, Rydholm A, Mitrelman M: Chromosomal abnormality t(9;22)(q22;q12) in an extraskeletal myxoid chondrosarcoma characterized by fine needle aspiration cytology, electron microscopy, immunohistochemistry and DNA flow cytometry. Cytopathology 1991;2:261–270.

134 Carlén B, Domanski HA, Mertens F, Åkerman M: Extraskeletal myxoid chondrosarcoma with neuroendocrine differentiation. Fine needle aspiration, histopathology, electron microscopy and cytogenetics. 1st Italian/Scandinavian Sarcoma Group Meeting-ISG/SSG. Acta Orthop Scand 2000;http://home.pi.se/actaorthopscand/pages/framabst.html.p33.

135 Folpe AL, Schmidt RA, Chapman A, Gown AM: Poorly differentiated synovial sarcoma: Immunohistochemical distinction from primitive neuroectodermal tumors and high grade malignant MPNST. Am J Surg Pathol 1998;22:673–682.

136 Kawai A, Woodruff J, Healy JH, Brennan MF, Antonescu CR, Ladanyi M: SYT-SSX gene fusion as a determinant of morphology and prognosis in synovial sarcoma. N Engl J Med 1998;338:153–160.

137 Nilsson G, Skytting B, Xie Y, Brodin B, Lundberg J, Uhlén M, Perfekt R, Mandahl N, Laresson O: The SYT-SSX1 variant of synovial sarcoma is associated with a high rate of tumor cell proliferation and poor clinical outcome. Cancer Res 1999;59:3180–3184.

138 Silverman JF, Landreneau RJ, Sturgis CD, Raab SS, Fox KR, Jasnosz KM, Dabbs DJ: Small-cell variant of synovial sarcoma: Fine-needle aspiration with ancillary features and potential diagnostic pitfalls. Diagn Cytopathol 2000;23:118–123.

139 Åkerman M, Ryd W, Skytting B: Fine needle aspiration of synovial sarcoma: Criteria for diagnosis: Retrospective reexamination of 37 cases, including ancillary diagnostics. A Scandinavian sarcoma group study. Diagn Cytopathol 2003;28:232–238.

Index